Concerning the Carers

Occupational Health for Health Care

Heinemann Medical

An imprint of Butterworth-Heinemann Ltd
Halley Court, Jordan Hill, Oxford OX2 8EJ

 PART OF REED INTERNATIONAL BOOKS

LONDON GUILDFORD OXFORD BOSTON SINGAPORE
SYDNEY TOKYO TORONTO WELLINGTON

First published 1991

British Library Cataloguing in Publication Data
Lunn, J. A.
  Concerning the carers : occupational health for health care
  workers.
  1. Welfare workers. Health
  I. Title II. Waldron, H. A. (Harry Arthur)
  363.15

  ISBN 0–7506–0022–5

Typeset by Lasertext Ltd., Stretford, Manchester
Printed and bound in Great Britain by Biddles Ltd, Guildford and
Kings Lynn

Contents

Preface

After many years of comparative neglect, occupational health provision for those working in the health services is now being given the attention it deserves. In the UK many units have been established in the last ten years or so but the effort has not been coordinated, nor have guidelines been issued on the best format which the individual services should take and there has been no attempt to ensure that standards and practices are uniform. In this book we are presenting our ideas, based on many years experience, of how best a service for health care workers can be set up and run.

We hope that all those who are actively engaged in running occupational health units in health services will find the book helpful and interesting. We would also like to think that other health care professionals will read it in order to inform themselves of the potential risks to which their work exposes them and the means by which some at least of these risks can be avoided. Since health and safety are nowadays rightly regarded as part of any manager's normal function, we hope that they too will find material in the book which gives them pause for thought.

There is a long tradition amongst those who care for others, of neglect of their own health; if this book goes some way to show that this is a tradition which has nothing to commend it and that they merit as much care as they provide for their patients, then we shall be satisfied.

J. A. Lunn and H. A. Waldron

CHAPTER 1

Introduction

By the very nature of most hospital and community health care work, automation is unlikely to lessen these services' almost total dependence on people for the provision of effective services to patients. The quality of the care and service which patients receive, depends not only on the calibre and professional expertise of the health care workers who provide that care, but also on the satisfactory maintenance of their health and general well-being.

Most multi-national companies and large industrial organizations have well-developed and coordinated occupational health services. The National Health Service is one of the largest employers in Europe, with over one million employees. It would not be an unreasonable assumption, that the NHS, because of its basic commitment to health, would be first and foremost in ensuring that its employees had the maximum health care, both curative and preventive. Unfortunately, as is often the case with doctors' and cobblers' families, the very reverse of this is at times true. The deficiencies in the occupational health provision were highlighted by Sir Ronald Tunbridge in 1968 in his report *The Care of the Health of Hospital Staff*. The report drew attention to the major defects in the provision of health care for workers in the hospital service. In the intervening years, a number of health authorities in England and Wales, and health boards in Scotland, have established occupational health services. The present Department of Health and former Department of Health and Social Security, has not established clear guidelines and standards on which to base occupational health services for the National Health Service as a whole. The Health and Safety Executive guidelines published in 1984 (see Appendix B) likewise are general in content and lack specific details. It has been left to individual health authorities and boards to decide how to make provision for protecting the health of their staff. Some authorities have been farseeing in establishing adequate services, while others have devoted the minimum of resources for occupational health services for their employees. The health authorities and boards in the UK which have established occupational health services have done so without there being a central and uniform standard for reference. The result has been that many of the services which have been developed have very varying standards, both in the calibre and qualifications of their professional staff, and also in the facilities and accommodation available.

The object of this book is to provide help and guidance to occupational health practitioners and to hospital personnel and managerial staff who have responsibilities for existing or future occupational health services for health care workers. Every hospital has its own specific problems and local requirements and it is not intended to suggest ways in which every aspect of an occupational health department should be run. It is intended, however, to indicate the general nature of the problems which need to be addressed and the important principles and standards which should be established. Some occupational health practitioners are concerned and uncertain about their roles and functions and find that these are not always adequately defined between doctor and nurse. We have been concerned to emphasize the tasks which require fulfilling and the qualifications and experience required to succeed. We do not believe that there can be any automatic assumption that the title of doctor or nurse fulfills a given role. We stress the importance of the professional competence and experience needed for the undertaking of all tasks in occupational health if adequate services are to be provided for health care workers, and if occupational health practitioners are to gain the respect of their fellow professionals in the other specialties in the health care services.

Medical and nursing staff who have had experience of working in more than one hospital or health authority will be aware of the variety of policies and clinical practices existing in the NHS for what should be essentially standard procedures. General control of infection and AIDS policies, for example, are almost as numerous and as varied as are the more than 200 health authorities and boards themselves, in spite of the fact that the problems to which the policies apply are virtually identical in each case. Occupational health practitioners may find themselves in difficult situations when their local professional committees advocate policies which conflict with those accepted in other health authorities and which occupational health practitioners have come to accept. Some local policies may also conflict with nationally, or internationally accepted practice, and indeed with recommendations — rare as they are — from the Department of Health. Whenever possible, we have made definitive recommendations for clinical practice and preventive procedures, so that the inexperienced reader is not presented with a variety of alternatives when faced with a situation in which only one course of action is possible. The recommendations made are based on a wide range of experience and occupational health practice in the health care field, for more than twenty years following the publication of the Tunbridge report in 1968.

It is of interest to note that during this near quarter of a century, there have been some significant changes and advances, notably in the field of infectious diseases and occupational risks from new therapies — lasers and cytotoxic drugs, for example. There is no longer the need for routine smallpox vaccinations, or for annual or indeed any routine chest X-rays. An effective vaccine against hepatitis B is now available and the virus responsible for AIDS has been identified although not mastered. Clinical practices in hospitals have changed greatly. Many surgical conditions at the beginning of this period were kept in hospital for 10-14 days postoperatively. Today, many of the same conditions are treated as day cases, or at least discharged within five days of operation.

This significant change has had a major effect on staff, mainly nursing. The much higher turnover of patients not only adds considerably to the intensity and pressure of work but also reduces the opportunity for staff to get to know their patients and to establish a satisfying professional relationship with them. This has not only added considerably to stress, but has also removed a great deal of job satisfaction. Morale, motivation, managerial attitudes and sickness absence have a close relationship. In discussing sickness absence, we have emphasized that organizational methods, managerial attitudes and lack of job satisfaction are as likely to play as important a part in influencing sickness absence rates as are any true fluctuations in the incidence of illness amongst staff. The ability to identify factors in the working environment which add to stress is important. It is also important that health care staff have the opportunity to be counselled when necessary, but as is emphasized later in the book, the counselling they receive must be adequate and professional. Many occupational health practitioners do not have the necessary counselling expertise and should not have a sense of failure if they find they have to refer cases to professionals with more adequate and appropriate training. To assist those who may not have the necessary expertise to deal with a wide range of problems requiring specialized knowledge and experience, a list of organizations and societies dealing with specific problems, either physical, psychological or addictive, is available in Appendix A.

Although occupational health is essentially a preventive discipline, it is appropriate to make some reference to the place of treatment, particularly in a hospital context. A number of conditions, mainly those of an infective nature, require early treatment not only for the benefit of the sufferer, but also to avoid the risk of infection to patients. In some cases, but for the latter concern, a number of conditions would not require treatment. It is not uncommon for there to be a delay of 4-5 days for an appointment to see a general practitioner, which is often an unacceptable time when infection control is important and in the meantime absence from work is necessary. Staff who have come to the hospital from other areas may not, at the time of being seen, have re-registered with a local general practitioner.

Early rehabilitation of staff with orthopaedic conditions may be aided by physiotherapy and provided there is adequate liaison with general practitioners, making this treatment available should also be considered. For these reasons occupational health practitioners should be aware of the benefits of providing treatment for health care workers in some circumstances.

ECONOMICS

Where health and well–being are concerned, it is difficult to justify every expense in terms of economic benefit. It is not easy to quantify the benefits of a contented and happy individual compared with an unhappy or depressed one, although the former is more likely to cope with caring and dealing with patients far more effectively than the latter. The number of cases of tuberculosis or hepatitis B prevented by comprehensive immunization programmes are not readily calculated. Indeed, the whole economics of health care provision would be hard to justify in purely materialistic terms and no one seriously seeks to do so. Nevertheless there are occasions when it is possible to point to clear financial benefits attributable to an occupational health unit. Where shortage of nursing staff results in ward closures, or the employment of large numbers of agency staff, significant reductions in sickness absence — which can be achieved by occupational health services — can represent at least an extra ward remaining open for a whole year.

MANAGERIAL RELATIONSHIPS

Occupational health practitioners have advisory and non-executive roles within their organizations. They must not assume or overlap any managerial functions of the hospital adminis-tration. It may at times be necessary to remind the management of the limitations imposed on an occupational health department by the nature of its advisory role. Unless management applies executive action to the advice it is given, the time and expertise of the occupational health department may be wasted.

It follows that there must be close liaison with management at all levels. The quality of the advice given and its constant impartiality will be the yardstick by which occupational health practitioners will be judged. By and large, changes in complex organizations will only be achieved by a quiet, restrained but competent approach. The special problems and sensitivities of every health care community must be understood before advocating change.

CHAPTER 2

Organization of occupational health services

ACCOMMODATION

In many hospitals there is often a serious shortage of space for acute medical services and adequate accommodation cannot be spared for an occupational health department. In newer buildings, including some large district hospitals, space for occupational health departments may not have been allocated in the planning stages and accommodation originally designed for other purposes is made available. For these reasons occupational health practitioners may sometimes find themselves working in accommodation not only limited in size but also which is placed at an unsuitable site in the hospital.

A number of occupational health departments within the NHS in the UK are providing services for district hospitals employing up to 5000 staff and in addition are providing a service for their local authority and other local employers. It is essential that adequate standards for occupational health accommodation are established to allow for provision not only for existing commitments within the hospital but also for commitments arising from the provision of additional services, especially for local authorities. It is not appropriate to suggest specific details or designs for departments as these are matters which only those acquainted with local problems and circumstances can decide. For those who have limited facilities or who are battling to avoid losing their existing accommodation some appropriate standards for accommodation for occupational health departments are outlined in Table 2.1.

It must be emphasized that the areas indicated are only general

TABLE 2.1

ACCOMMODATION FOR OCCUPATIONAL HEALTH DEPARTMENTS

	Area	
	sq ft	sq m
Reception, secretarial, current records	180	17
Record storage	100	10
Waiting room	100	10
Treatment and immunization	200	21
Occupational health doctor	140	13
Occupational health nursing adviser 1	140	13
Occupational health nursing adviser 2	140	13
Rest room	140	13
Toilets and urine testing space	40	4
	1180	114

guidelines and not rigid indications of what must be established. The space advocated will allow for adequate occupational health services for most district hospitals and also for expansion of the service to cover local authority and other commitments. There may be little choice over where the accommodation is sited within the hospital but strong pleas should be made to avoid it being placed next door to personnel or nursing administration offices or other similar havens of management and authority. Ideally the department should be in an approachable but quiet part of the hospital which is not unduly exposed to public scrutiny. This will encourage members of staff to attend who might be deterred if they had to do so with the certainty of public observation.

MANAGEMENT

Occupational health practitioners may at times experience difficulties in establishing the management roles and responsibilities of their departments. There is an extremely wide range of professional experience and qualifications amongst doctors and nurses who practice occupational health within the NHS in the UK. The ability of any given individual to manage and advise on the various aspects of the running of a department will differ considerably from one hospital to another. Some of the more important issues will be outlined and after considering these occupational health practitioners may find their managerial problems more easily resolved.

The occupational health department is by and large comparable, as far as general organization is concerned, to many other departments within a hospital. It is therefore important to conform as far as possible to the general style and standards of the overall organization and not to seek unnecessary variations. It is not necessary to insist on the person who is ultimately responsible for professional standards having responsibility for the day–to–day organization and running of the department or for the financial commitments. Not all higher training courses in occupational health give consideration to management and budgetary aspects of occupational health and a higher qualification should not necessarily imply the possession of this competence.

Most nursing practitioners have considerable experience of organizing and running departments even before they specialize in occupational health. It is recommended that those most experienced in general management and budgeting should have responsibility for those aspects of the department. There may be more difficulty when matters concerning the personnel of the department arise. Each profession has its own background experience and expertise and it is probably not conducive to good professional relationships to have one profession responsible for another and therefore it is recommended that the nursing and medical staff do not have cross accountability for each other. Responsibility for the professional policies and standards of a department must ultimately be that of the most experienced and qualified occupational health practitioner. It must be stressed however that on occasions both medical and nursing staff are appointed to occupational health posts in hospitals where neither has adequate experience or qualifications of the speciality. In these circumstances it would be inappropriate for either practitioner to be the ultimate arbiter of professional policy and it is strongly recommended that those in this position should consult their more experienced and qualified colleagues in other hospitals.

CONFIDENTIALITY

Some of the older members of the nursing profession will be able to recall the occasions during their training when they could seek medical advice only from one nominated doctor in the hospital and always, without choice, in the presence of the home sister. However undesirable this arrangement may have been, it did at least have an open frankness about it which left no one in any doubt where they stood. Some present-day arrangements for dealing with medical information about health care workers are not always as confidential as they may appear to be.

It is the responsibility of occupational health practitioners to establish, maintain and monitor confidential record systems and procedures and to ensure that the managements of their organizations respect these arrangements. In hospitals and community clinics it is essential that occupational health notes and records are kept quite separately from any clinical case notes which may be established for employees who are treated as ordinary patients in the hospital in which they work. If medical staff who are seeing them in these circumstances request to see the occupational health notes for additional information to help them deal with a clinical problem they must be advised that only a relevant summary of the notes can be given provided written consent is given by the employee.

Occupational records must never leave occupational health departments except when being transferred to another unit within the same service. Pre-employment health questionnaires must be marked confidential to the occupational health department. It is not unknown for personnel departments and employing managers to issue the health questionnaires to prospective employees and to receive the completed forms themselves before they are sent on to the occupational health department. This is wrong practice and should never happen. All health questionnaires should be issued with envelopes marked 'confidential' and addressed to the occupational health department for direct return when completed.

Forms used to notify the management that an applicant is fit or not for employment should not contain medical details but only the interpretation of any medical condition in terms of the applicant's ability to undertake the proposed employment. This principle applies equally when a report is given to management about an employee who has been referred for assessment because of a recurrent sickness absence pattern or after one particular spell of sickness.

When employees are involved in litigation regarding their

health and employment, management may ask to see occupational health records as of assumed right. The records must not be released under these circumstances unless an employee gives written permission or unless there is a specific legal requirement to do so. Some managers find it difficult to accept that they do not have an automatic right to see their staff's occupational health records and sometimes marked pressure is placed on occupational health practitioners to release records in cases of litigation. It is always essential to adhere to the correct policies on confidentiality in these circumstances.

Ethical Considerations

There are circumstances where the safety and well-being of patients and other staff, require that an employee should not remain at work — open pulmonary tuberculosis, enteric and skin infections, and some psychiatric illnesses including drug addiction, for example. If an employee will not accept the need to be away from work while appropriate treatment is received, the occupational health practitioner will be obliged to inform the management that the employee is unfit to remain at work. Before this is done, the employee and trade union representative if available, should be fully advised of the action which must be taken.

Records

An almost infinite variety of record systems exists within occupational health departments of the hospital services in the UK. It is likely that the majority of these systems perform an adequate function within the limited circumstances in which they are used. Those who use the records and who may have designed and developed them will probably be convinced that their systems are at least as good and probably better than any other. Many occupational health practitioners develop the pride of parenthood for their documentary innovations and become extremely sensitive to any criticism, however gently made or justified.

The wider the variety of record systems in existence the more difficult it is to coordinate research projects, epidemiological studies and the exchange of records when individuals transfer from one hospital to another. Medical records and forms on the whole reflect fairly closely the policies and standards of those who use them. Health questionnaires used for pre-employment screening illustrate this point well. Many contain questions which have little or no relevance on deciding on fitness for health care work or any other occupation. The presence of irrelevant questions inevitably raises doubts about the criteria being applied for assessing fitness to work by those using the form. The absence of some questions may be of equal significance. There should be consistent standards of fitness for health care workers for comparable occupations. Health questionnaires should therefore reflect a uniform standard for selecting applicants for employment and be similar in their content.

It is important to ensure that completed health questionnaires are returned directly to the occupational health department and pre-printed envelopes marked confidential to the occupational health department should be sent out with each questionnaire. Some record systems, although containing a mass of information, do not allow the information to be readily accessible — for example where details of immunizations are written on separate pages which are widely dispersed throughout the medical records. This does not give an opportunity for an instant appraisal of the immunization state of an individual. It is recommended that basic occupational health information about employees which is not essentially confidential should be stored in appropriately separated sections. This will enable basic information to be readily transferred from one place of employment to another and avoid tests and investigations being needlessly repeated. It is perhaps worth emphasizing that however well designed a record system is, its ultimate effectiveness will depend on the accuracy of recording and filing of documents.

Another aspect of documentation is the need for it to be clear and simple and easily understood by those receiving it. This particularly applies to forms notifying personnel or managers about an applicant's fitness for work. Sometimes these forms have such a multiplicity of detail on them attempting to cover every eventuality that it is not clear what the message is. It is recommended that eventualities which may arise only once or twice a year should not be included. Such events should be dealt with on a 'one-off' basis by letter on the occasions on which they occur. In general a good style of documentation should be established and it should not be left to every individual in one organization to create their own forms without regard to this. Each form should have a code reference to identify its origin and should display the proper title of the health authority and hospital from which it originates. It is important to date all documents so that when they are revised the old versions can be readily identified.

MEMBERSHIP OF COMMITTEES

Occupational health practitioners have only advisory roles to management and no executive authority. In order to play an effective advisory role there must be adequate dialogue with management and staff. One way in which this can be achieved is by adequate representation on appropriate committees such as control of infection, health and safety and radiological safety committees. Occupational health practitioners should also be represented on committees of senior nursing management and medical committees within their own hospitals. There should also be representation on all working groups on which staff health issues are being discussed. When smoking and alcohol policies are being considered and planned for example, it is essential that occupational health practitioners are part of those working groups. Often misunderstandings about the role of occupational health exist among management and staff. Each side may suspect that occupational health is biased towards the other and as a result occupational health independence may not be fully accepted or understood.

There is much to recommend the establishment of an occupational health steering committee with representatives from all sides of hospital employment. This committee can act as an ideal forum for correcting misunderstandings and exchanging information and as a means of keeping in close touch with employee and management issues. This type of committee is not generally established, often because there has been anxiety that it might interfere with the independence of the occupational health department. If properly constituted and constructively used the steering committee can be of great value in furthering the function and aims of occupational health.

HEALTH EDUCATION

It is recommended that all occupational health departments establish an information board on which is displayed current information on health and safety issues and safety equipment. These boards may be placed either in the waiting room or outside the main entrance to the department. In addition to this, it is suggested that general health education pamphlets, obtainable from health education departments, should also be displayed in racks. There is a wide variety of these, ranging from 'healthy eating' to various aspects of disease prevention. It is also recommended that the occupational health department should act as a general source of information for staff in other areas which are not strictly occupational. For example, it is helpful to have a list of local family planning clinics, and their times, and whether or not these require appointments to be made. Likewise, clinics providing cervical cytology and 'well-woman' facilities should be indicated, together with lists of local general medical and dental practitioners. Some hospitals provide dental and chiropody services within the hospital, and where these facilities are available, it is important that staff are adequately informed about them and the arrangements for making appointments.

THE PROVISION OF OCCUPATIONAL HEALTH SERVICES TO NON-HEALTH CARE WORKERS

For many years some hospital occupational health departments have provided a service to their local authorities. Recently however, there has been a tendency to expand these developments to provide additional occupational health services not only to local authority employees but to those of other industries. In some areas local authority employees attend the hospital occupational health unit and no specific provision is made at the local authority premises. In other cases full occupational health clinics are established in the civic centres, staffed by full-time occupational health nurses and a part-time doctor, and these staff may either be directly employed by the local or by the hospital authority.

In the interests of developing coordinated policies it may be helpful for all the occupational health staff to be employed by the hospital authority and the relevant costs charged to the local authority. Where there has been some rudimentary occupational health service already in existence in the local authority there will be a medical record system in existence. In this situation there is the possibility that two record systems may run side by side and whenever possible it is strongly recommended that one uniform record system is established.

PROVISION OF OCCUPATIONAL HEALTH SERVICES FOR PRIVATE CONTRACTORS

A considerable number of hospitals in the NHS have contracted out their domestic and catering services to private firms who recruit and employ their own labour. In the majority of instances in which this has happened it has been agreed that the existing occupational health services of these hospitals will provide a service for the outside contractors.

The primary importance of this arrangement is the guarantee it gives to the hospitals concerned that the same standards of medical selection will apply to the contractors' employees. It also ensures that immunization and control of infection policies will be applied. Some occupational health services have experienced difficulties in establishing adequate liaison with the managements of outside contractors due as a rule to their lack of experience of hospital requirements rather than to any positive intentions not to cooperate. The establishment of a hospital liaison manager may improve communications and cooperation.

Whenever occupational health practitioners in the hospital service provide cover for private contractors it is important to have clear written statements about the extent of the occupational health cover to be provided. When the cover is limited to pre-employment health screening, immunization and post-employment monitoring for infection risks, it is important to ensure that the contractors' managers understand the significance of the limited cover being provided. This will mean, for example, that the service provided will not deal with problems such as back pain in their staff or the problems of fitness to work after long-term illness, unless issues of infection control are involved.

The financial arrangements for providing occupational health services to outside contractors are varied and some hospital managements make no charge for the service provided, arguing that to do so would in turn raise the overall charges made by the contractors for their services. An important point which may need to be emphasized to hospital management is the disproportionate demand made on occupational health resources by some outside contractors because of the high turnover of their staff. Many catering firms have an annual staff turnover rate of over 100%. This must be taken into account when the amount of work is being assessed. The total number of staff employed by the contractor at any one time will not as a rule adequately indicate the amount of work created for the department.

CHAPTER 3

Staffing of occupational health services

In any occupational health service the number and type of staff is determined to a large extent by the perceived hazards to which the workforce are exposed, by the care and concern shown by management towards those whom they employ, by any legal requirements and by economic constraints. Working in the health care professions is not generally perceived to be a high–risk occupation, the care and concern shown by the most senior management (not excluding various health ministers and their officials) has never been overwhelming and there are few legal constraints which have to be observed. It comes as no surprise therefore, to find that the provision of occupational health services for those who care for others has come late, is often inadequate and frequently held in low esteem by colleagues in other disciplines.

In fact there is plenty of evidence to suggest that health care work has been and continues to be a risky business. There is a tendency to think that the risks attached to the work are only of historical interest and to ignore the chemical, physical and psychological hazards with which it abounds. In fact, the need for occupational health services to be set up in the NHS was recognised by the Tunbridge Committee as long ago as 1968 but it is only in the last twenty years that health authorities have made any real effort to provide them.

PRESENT PROVISIONS

The present provision of occupational health services within the NHS in the UK could perhaps be most kindly described as haphazard. The Department of Health has never been seen strenuously to support occupational health services for its staff, still less to attempt to set up a national service with consistent standards, policies and work practices. Each health authority has, therefore, tended to go it alone and so those services which are now in place take many forms. The one thing which they almost all have in common is that they are nurse–based; that is to say, the majority of the staff are nurses who do most of the day–to–day work. The medical support may come from local general practitioners on a sessional basis; from senior clinical medical officers; from clinical assistants or other part-time doctors who may be working in other areas of occupational health; from private consultants; or from consultant occupational physicians who may or may not be full-time. In some services the doctor is the director of the service and the budget holder although without necessarily managing the service. Elsewhere, the manager and budget holder is a nurse. Some departments have nurses in training and a much smaller number have registrar or senior registrar posts which are almost always jointly funded with a local industrial concern. The majority of full-time staff, however, do have some formal qualification in occupational health.

Very few departments employ an occupational hygienist or a safety officer but rather more have the services of psychiatrists, psychologists, physiotherapists and all, of course, have clerical and secretarial help.

STAFFING LEVELS

It is almost impossible to be dogmatic about the number of staff of the various grades that are required by an occupational health department within the health service. However, as a rough rule of thumb it would be reasonable to have occupational health nurse advisers in the ratio of one per one or two thousand employees. It is likely that one medical session would be needed for each thousand employees. The question of who should be manager of the service is discussed elsewhere (*see* Chapter 2); suffice it to say here that it would be difficult for anyone to manage a sizeable occupational health service unless he or she were employed in a full-time capacity.

To what extent the services of other professionals are needed is very much a matter of local need. Several units do have sessions from specialists in musculo-skeletal disorders (who may be doctors or physiotherapists) specifically to deal with back injuries and to teach proper lifting and handling techniques; some offer counselling services to staff and in others, psychiatrists come in for one or two sessions a month to advise staff who have psychiatric illnesses. Those departments which do have help from other disciplines are generally enthusiastic about the benefits which accrue to them from the presence of a large multi-disciplinary team but in only a few cases is any formal audit or cost-benefit analysis undertaken; it is sometimes difficult not to harbour the suspicion that size rather than efficacy is the criterion by which some managers judge the success of their department.

One trend which needs particularly careful supervision is that towards offering counselling services to staff. Stress is often perceived as a serious occupational hazard for health care workers and is frequently cited as the reason for work withdrawal, for failure to complete training and for a high turnover rate. Although it may not always be possible to cite data in support of these contentions, nevertheless, experience teaches that some areas of clinical work — dealing with children with malignant disease, for example — are particularly stressful, and the stringencies within which the health service has now to work, impose considerable stress upon all managers.

Occupational health departments, and especially some occupational health nurse advisers are seeing it as their function to provide counselling services for employees, either singly or in groups. It is at least questionable whether occupational health departments should be the providers of such a service; two matters are of particular concern, the qualifications of those offering the counselling and their supervision. It should be an absolute rule that occupational health staff (and that includes *all* staff) should not enter into therapeutic counselling unless they have adequate formal training and preferably hold a recognized qualification. Even though these criteria are fulfilled, it is essential that staff who provide a counselling service are properly supervised by someone outside the department with the necessary experience and qualifications. Counselling is not just an extension of tea and sympathy and the sooner this is understood the better.

In the view of the authors, the occupational health department does best by acting as a facilitator for counselling, and a wide range of other peripheral services. It seems perfectly proper that members of staff should see the occupational health department as their point of contact when they have a problem and that the members of the department should offer what help they can in the short-term and at the same time make an assessment as to the best course of action in the long-term; this might well include referral to an outside counselling agency, one with which the occupational health department had some contact and in which they had confidence.

Personnel

Occupational health practice is a team affair, but to be effective, it is important to recruit the right team. The predominant role will continue to be taken by occupational health nurse advisers but they should be supported wherever possible by an occupational physician of consultant status. The importance of having consultants in occupational health departments is that they have access to the committees at which policy and funding decisions are taken and they also have an equal standing with their other medical colleagues. One difficulty which occupational health departments are experiencing at present is attracting men or women of the right quality into consultant posts. Since there are at present few opportunities to train junior staff in occupational health departments there is no ready stream of senior registrars able to take up consultant posts and very few industrial medical officers seem to want to make the move into the health service. This is a matter which needs some urgent consideration by the Department of Health; we allude to this again below. One solution might be to create consultant posts jointly with industry so that the incumbent would spend time partly in the health service and partly in industry.

The core personnel will be supported by clerical and secretarial staff. To what extent it will be necessary to have other categories of staff will depend upon the nature of the risks at work and this will only be brought to light by analysis of attendance registers or by special surveys. Back pain is almost always likely to be an important cause of morbidity and time lost from work and it is extremely helpful if one of the medical staff has, or can work up, some interest and expertise in the area of musculo-skeletal training and rehabilitation. Where the problem is extreme, employing a physiotherapist should easily be shown to be cost-effective. Following the implementation of the Control of Substances Hazardous to Health (COSHH) Regulations, occupational health departments are increasingly involved in work place assessments which may more properly be seen to be within the remit of an occupational hygienist rather than a nurse or a physician. Very few departments could justify taking on an occupational hygienist, however, if only because the cost of equipping a hygiene laboratory would be well beyond their means. However, it may well be that a hygienist could be employed on a regional basis, or shared with a local industry, or with a local academic department (if there are any left). It may be possible to hire out the services of such an individual to other concerns which also needed to make assessments to comply with the regulations but had no need for a full-time hygienist.

One of the most important functions of the occupational health department, however, is not to employ a wide variety of professionals but to develop a network of contacts who can either be used on an *ad hoc* basis or to whom members of staff can be referred on for a second opinion or for assessment and treatment. A close working relationship with psychiatrists, psychologists, dermatologists and rheumatologists is essential to deal with the common work-related problems which arise. A liaison with endocrinologists and neurologists might also be desirable if there is a positive policy to accept for training those who have either insulin dependent diabetes or epilepsy. Some ready means of referral to agencies which will deal with alcoholism, stress and obesity will also prove beneficial.

Training

To attract, recruit and retain individuals of high calibre into occupational medicine or occupational nursing requires the provision of proper training and it has to be said that it is by no means adequate at present.

Occupational nurses will require the Occupational Health Nursing Diploma (which has recently been upgraded from the Occupational Health Nursing Certificate) if they wish to progress far in their career and there are many part-time or full-time courses which serve as a preparation for the examination.

Generally there is no difficulty in arranging for attendance at part-time courses but almost no provision for full-time training. It is important for at least one post in a large occupational health department to be a training post and this seems to be generally accepted.

The provision of training for potential occupational physicians, however, is another matter. For the purposes of specialist accreditation, the Faculty of Occupational Medicine requires that some post-graduate training takes place at senior registrar level and there are precious few such posts at present. The post must be recognized by the Faculty and the tendency has been to consider that experience solely within the health service is not adequate and this is why most posts are a joint venture between the health service and industry. This attitude should change in the future as more and more occupational health departments in the health service begin to provide a service to outside agencies, including small industries.

It is regrettable that the Deparment of Health does not see fit to provide a substantial number of senior registrar posts since if it does not, then it is hard to see where the consultants of the future are to come from; having said that, there is certainly no prospect of any change and those who presently hold consultant posts must accept it as their responsibility to go through the time-consuming and rather thankless task of persuading their Regional Health Authority to create new posts. There is also the not inconsiderable hurdle to be overcome of finding the money for their salaries. Nevertheless, the importance of training to the development, or even the continuance, of occupational health as a discipline within the health service cannot be stressed enough and all practitioners must see it as a fundamental part of their work. Since it is likely that the service will need to depend on the part-time doctors — be they general practitioners or others — for the foreseeable future, it is equally important that their training needs are also met so the quality can be maintained. The training requirements for all staff, then, must be considered when estimating the training budget.

CHAPTER 4

Selection of staff as health care workers

If anyone unconnected with occupational health were to be asked how its practitioners spend their time, there is a high probability that pre-employment medical assessment would figure high on the list. And traditionally this has been the case. Indeed it was not so long ago that a great deal of the occupational physician's week was taken up with the examination of applicants for jobs with little or no benefit to the employer, the candidate for the post or to the physician. Increasingly the role of pre-employment health assessment has been called into question and some of the issues will be examined in this chapter and some approaches will be suggested which may have more to commend them than those which have been followed in the past.

THE FUNCTION OF PRE-EMPLOYMENT HEALTH SCREENING

It is important to remember that there are three parties involved in pre-employment health screening and that their interests do not necessarily coincide. First, the employer. It is implicit (and sometimes explicit) in the employer's attitude to pre-employment screening that it should serve the purpose of ensuring that only healthy people are taken into work and that there is a reasonable prospect that they will continue in this state of good health for the foreseeable future; or at least for five years when they will be likely to change jobs. It is difficult not to have some sympathy with this point of view especially when faced with high turnover rates, difficulties in recruiting and keeping staff, high sickness absence rates and the costs involved in training. On the matter of accepting men or women for training, whether as nurses or as doctors, there is the additional concern that for each candidate who fails to complete the course for reasons of ill health, another (who might have finished) has been rejected; thus a sense of double obligation is sometimes felt by those making the selection, both towards those whom they accept and those whom they reject.

For those looking for a job or a place on a course, however, the matter is completely different. Their over-riding anxiety is to get accepted and the health interview, or medical examination is most often seen as an inconvenient hurdle standing in their way. It is possible, therefore, that some applicants will be somewhat economical with the truth when replying either to a questionnaire or to direct questioning from a member of the occupational health staff and it has to be said, that their medical advisers may sometimes collude with them if they see this as serving the best interests of their patients.

In the middle stands the honest broker; the occupational health professional whose responsibility is to ensure the best possible fit between the individual and the position which he or she is hoping to occupy.

How is it Done?

There are three principal levels of pre-employment health assessment;

1. complete medical examination
2. questionnaire augmented by an interview with an occupational health nurse
3. reliance solely on questionnaire.

Most departments would recognize their own practice as falling within one or other of these categories.

Most practitioners are agreed that medical examination of all prospective new employees or candidates for training posts within the health service has nothing whatever to commend it and that it is a practice to be discouraged wherever it still lingers on unless the circumstances are exceptional.

Screening by questionnaire is almost certainly the most

commonly used form of pre-employment health assessment and a huge number of questionnaires has been devised over the years. None is altogether satisfactory, but most units have evolved one which suits their purpose. The health service does not have a uniform questionnaire which could be used by all occupational health units but a working party convened by the Department of Health and the Health and Safety Executive is in the process of producing a suggested format for discussion. In the meantime, some individual occupational health units are collaborating to produce one for themselves. If this form of screening is to continue, it is desirable that the forms used by occupational health departments should be standardized so that some consistency in practice can be achieved throughout the health service.

The procedure which is usually followed is that applicants complete the form as best they can and return it direct to the occupational health department. To avoid unnecessary work, it is preferable that only candidates who are being seriously considered for a post be asked to complete the form but this is often not the case.

Once in the department the forms are scanned by the occupational health nurse who should make one of three decisions; to advise that the candidate is fit for the post; to decide that more information is required; or to refer the form to the occupational physician. It is an absolute rule that only the physician can take the decision that a candidate is medically unsuited for a post. It is obvious, that in order to determine an individual's fitness for a post, those who are making the decision must be familiar with the physical and mental demands of the job and with any special risks which are inherent in it. This cannot be achieved without constant forays onto the shop floor and it must be emphasized that the hospital or clinic is a work-place like any other and it is just as important to keep the working environment under review as it is the workforce.

With some questionnaires it may not be possible for the nurse immediately to arrive at a definite conclusion. This may be because there is too little information or too much. Some candidates feel obliged to be circumstantial and over-inclusive so that each tiny skin blemish is described at length and each attack of upper respiratory infection is minutely detailed whereas others may answer 'No' to a question which asks if they have had any serious illnesses in the past, omitting the fact that they were in hospital for eight months with a psychotic depression. The latter are rather more difficult to deal with than the former. When faced with an equivocal questionnaire, the nurse may feel that she requires further details or clarification on some points and it was not unusual in the past to write to the individual's own general practitioner to request this information. Since the *Access to Medical Information Act* of 1988, however, doctors may not give such information without the patient's permission and the patient has up to 21 days in which to see a report before it is sent. This has tended to change practice in two ways; firstly, the request is addressed to the individual much more frequently than was formerly the case and secondly, the nurse making the assessment tends to refer to the physician rather more than in the past.

Referral to the physician results either in an acceptance on the basis of the questionnaire with or without supplementary information, or in a consultation. Following the consultation, the physician may consider the candidate fit, fit subject to certain restrictions, or unfit. Exceptionally it may be possible to engage a candidate on a short-term contract (say for six months) with a review at the end; this is sometimes referred to as 'a trial of labour'. No candidate can be turned down without an interview and without being told the reasons why he or she is considered medically unsuitable. This can be an extremely unpleasant and often distressing experience for both the doctor and the candidate but must never be shirked by the practitioner on this account.

The third approach to pre-employment screening is that of a questionnaire supplemented by a health assessment with an occupational health nurse. In order for this to be cost-effective it is necessary that only candidates who have had a job offer are seen and the degree of collaboration between the personnel and occupational health departments required to run such a system effectively and efficiently is not always forthcoming. The rationale of the interview is that it is possible to get a much better impression of health and fitness than from a questionnarie alone. For some occupations — and catering is the most obvious example — it is clearly preferable to screening by questionnaire alone. The interview itself can be augmented by other procedures; for example, measuring spinal mobility in those whose work involves lifting or examining the skin and performing lung function tests on those who might come into contact with a sensitizer such as formaldehyde, glutaraldehyde or experimental animals.

Routine Chest X-Rays

Until comparatively recently it was customary to ask each applicant for a post in the health service to have a chest X-Ray unless they could produce a satisfactory report on one which had been carried out within the past year. The reason for this was to contain the spread of tuberculosis from staff to patients or to other members of staff. There is nothing now to commend this practice although we note that some units still adhere rigidly to it.

Current thinking, however, is that no-one should be subjected to ionizing radiation unnecessarily and a chest X-ray should be requested only when there is a clinical indication for so doing; this is the basis of good clinical practice in any event, and should always have been so. The prevalence of tuberculosis amongst the indigenous population in the UK is now such that the likelihood of detecting an asymptomatic case of the disease by routine chest X-ray is so low as to render it a futile exercise, even if no other consideration were to be taken into account. (As an aside, it should be noted that several thousands of pounds could be saved by abandoning this arcane practice and this is no small consideration in these cost conscious days.) It *is* a requirement, however, that all staff who regularly come into patient contact or who regularly enter clinical areas or who handle potentially infected material should be immune to tuberculosis and this issue is discussed in more detail in chapter 7.

Which Form of Pre-employment Assessment

Certainly the most cost-effective method of pre-employment screening is by health questionnaire alone. It is doubtful whether the results obtained from routine health interview justify the extra time and effort involved; it is taken as read that no-one would wish to undertake medical examinations as a routine. Within the health service, however, the majority of the applicants for jobs and certainly the overwhelming majority of candidates for training are young; in one of our units the outcome of pre-employment assessments was monitored for six months and the average age of the applicants for jobs (not trainees) was 28.5 years (with a range from 17–54; the oldest person was applying for a post as an elderly care adviser). Almost 92 % of applicants were accepted; further information was sought on 7 % none of whom was referred to the occupational physician although a further 8 % were referred to the physician on the basis of information in the questionnaire. Overall, the rejection rate was 3 %.

Although these are preliminary data from a single unit they suggest that the system for health assessment might be changed. One way might be simply to target the population most at risk and restrict any form of health assessment to those over 40 or 50; the lower age limit could be determined actuarily if necessary. In these days of equal opportunities, however, such an approach might be condemned as being 'ageist'; we would, therefore, like to consider other methods.

The Job-Risk Profile

The objective of the pre-employment health assessment is, as has been said, to ensure that all individuals are fit to carry out the job or the training for which they have applied. Two factors need to be considered; firstly, contrary to what most managers might think, it is not necessary to be healthy to work, only that the state of health does not impair the capacity to carry out a particular job and that it is not likely that the condition will be the cause of frequent sickness absence. Secondly, the special requirements of the job must be known and to that end, a risk-profile of the occupations within the health service can be drawn up with the aid of the managers of each of the departments concerned.

To compile a risk profile, the day-to-day activities in each job category must be known in some detail and the managers should be asked to say what conditions they consider to be inimical to each job. It is the task of the occupational health department finally to compile the risk-profile but ultimately it is managers who must determine who they will or will not accept to work in their departments so long as they stay within the law and so it is vital that they are directly involved with the procedure; this is in line with current thinking in which the prime responsibility for health and safety is seen to rest firmly with management and not with the occupational health department.

The compilation of risk-profiles for all categories of staff within the health service will not be achieved without considerable effort and to date little work has been carried out in this area, although both the occupational nurses and the occupational physicians have issued some guidance for selecting applicants for nurse training.

We have looked at the position with respect to applicants for nurse training where the special occupational risks are from back pain and dermatitis, especially affecting the hands. Levels of stress are also acknowledged to be high and at least one recent study has shown them to be higher in nurses than in other health care professionals. There is also the risk which they share with other health care workers of contracting infectious diseases from their patients.

What medical conditions would we consider to be an absolute bar to accepting a candidate for nurse training? Those which relate to their special risks include contact dermatitis which affects the skin and which requires constant treatment to keep it under control; a history of frequent back pain which has necessitated losing time from work or from school or college; serious psychiatric disorders including anorexia nervosa or any psychotic illness such as schizophrenia or psychotic depression unless there has been at least two years without symptoms; any condition in which there is suppression of the immune response including that induced by drug treatment.

There are in addition a few other conditions which would disbar a candidate for nurse training or at least cause them to defer their application for a year or two. These include uncontrolled epilepsy in which the individual has had fits during the last two years during waking hours whether or not on medication; brittle or uncontrolled insulin-dependent diabetes; complete deafness and some physical disabilities which impair movement or dexterity.

With the risk profile to hand and agreed with management, then there are two options. The usual health questionnaire can be sent out to applicants, returned and scanned and those who admit of conditions which are a bar to acceptance rejected, with or without seeing the physician depending on how clear cut the evidence is from the questionnaire and any supplementary details. Alternatively, a form can be sent which lists those conditions which would disqualify an applicant for the job they are seeking, with reasons; the circumstances under which an application is best deferred; and, importantly, those conditions which are acceptable. Candidates would then be asked to return to the occupational health department (or the the personnel department since confidentiality is not an issue here) a simple statement to the effect that they have read the document and that they have none of the conditions which would disbar them from the post in question. It would have to be made clear that if they were found to have any of the proscribed conditions once they had started work, this would result in their suspension and perhaps their dismissal and they might wish to discuss the form with their own medical adviser before returning the signed statement.

Clearly the health service is a long way from adopting such an approach and we have no doubt that some of our nursing and medical colleagues would not be in favour of such radical change. However it is an approach which merits further research and evaluation. There is a tendency towards inertia within many occupational health units, and research and audit are not prominent amongst their activities. This somewhat complacent attitude must change if the speciality is to remain viable.

Movement Within the Health Service

One of the most absurd features of occupational health practice within the health service is that staff who move from one hospital to another are more often than not required to undergo a health assessment before their new post is confirmed. Staff who choose to stay where they are for twenty or thirty years are, naturally, never put to this inconvenience. In some instances, Heaf or Mantoux tests are repeated although this is undesirable (*see* chapter 7). Some units do request information from the occupational health department at the last place of work but this is not always forthcoming. It would be much simpler and much more satisfactory if at least those parts of the records which gave details of immunization, sickness absences, accidents at work and the original health questionnaire could be transferable.

There may well be clinical details which individuals would prefer were kept confidential to the person to whom they were originally divulged but it should not be difficult to devise a scheme which allowed the ready transfer of non-sensitive information.

Informing Management of Outcome

Whatever form of pre-employment health assessment is used, it is essential that the result is relayed quickly (that is within 24 or 48 hours) to the personnel department or the the departmental manager. It is easiest to use a standard form for this purpose which will show either that the individual is fit for the post for which he or she has applied; fit subject to the restrictions which are indicated; or unfit. If further information is required, or if a consultation is necessary, the form should say this and indicate that a final result will follow as soon as possible.

Where time is of the essence, the result may be given on the telephone but the verbal message *must* be confirmed in writing, preferably on the same day.

Follow up of Staff after Employment

All new members of staff should be seen in the occupational health department as soon as possible after they start. The reasons for this include firstly to ensure that those who may be at risk from infection are properly immunized; secondly so that work practices and emergency procedures — such as the reporting of sharps injuries — can be explained; and finally in order to try to ensure that each new member of staff is aware of the functions and responsibilities of the occupational health department and how best they can use it. Some departments have developed a folder or booklet which outlines their duties and responsibilities, including opening hours and telephone numbers and this is often found to be extremely helpful.

Routine Health Surveillance

Until recently there was no requirement for any staff in the health service to undergo routine health surveillance although those exposed to X-ray irradiation were obliged to wear film badges to monitor the dose which they received. It was also recommended that staff in laboratories handling pathogens should be seen annually and have annual chest X-rays but there will certainly be a change in policy regarding the latter. Other departments have chosen to monitor other categories of staff on an *ad hoc* basis; for example, it is commonplace that hospital drivers are examined every year and for staff in animal houses to have annual lung function tests. With the advent of the Control of Substances Hazardous to Health (COSHH) Regulations, which came in to force in October 1989, however, the position has changed somewhat.

The regulations require that all work which involves exposure to substances hazardous to health, both chemical and biological, must be assessed in order to determine the risks to employees and the measures which must be taken in order to minimize them. There may be a call for environmental monitoring in some circumstances if it seems likely that exposures in excess of the the occupational exposure limit can occur and there is also a requirement for regular health surveillance where this is considered necessary.

There are not likely to be many circumstances under which monitoring or health surveillance will be required except where there is exposure to those substances which are thought to be the most hazardous. These include sensitizers such as glutaraldehyde, formaldehyde and experimental animals, anaesthetic gases, cytotoxic drugs, mercury, solvents such as xylene, toluene and white spirit and ethylene oxide.

These substances are considered in more detail in chapter 5, but suffice it to say here, that the occupational health department should at least compile registers of members of staff exposed to these substances. In the case of sensitizers an initial screen is almost certainly likely to be seen as a requirement as part of the initial assessment and some environmental monitoring will be required where the conditions under which solvents are used seem unsatisfactory and in operating theatres or recovery rooms where ventilation is inadequate.

The COSHH regulations will inevitably generate more work for occupational health departments but they should also help to bring health and safety much more to the fore than has previously been the case and occupational health professionals ought to welcome this opportunity to enhance their own standing.

CHAPTER 5

Infectious, chemical and some other hazards

Working in the health care professions carries with it a number of risks although it is perhaps reassuring that at least some of those involved enjoy a better than average expectation of life. For example, the standardized mortality ratios (SMRs) for doctors in the UK are 81 (for males) and 68 (for females); for nurses the SMR is 96. On the down side, however, it should be noted that SMRs for some particular causes of death are extremely high; thus for suicide and for alcohol related diseases they are 311 and 335 respectively. Both may be related to stress although the reason for the high suicide rate has also to do with the fact that health professionals generally have a better than average understanding of how to go about it, and also have relatively ready access to the means of procuring their own death.

There are a number of hazards which are shared by a majority of those working in a health service, particularly the risk of infection both from direct contact with patients or with potentially infected specimens or instruments. Certain groups of staff have special risks which arise directly from their work and, as in most other industries, these risks may be chemical, biological or physical. In this chapter and the next the most important of these are discussed and the risks set into perspective and ways of minimizing the risks and monitoring those exposed to them are suggested.

INFECTIOUS DISEASE

Staff in hospitals and other clinical settings are potentially at risk of contracting many infectious diseases directly from patients or from the handling or preparation of infected specimens or instruments. The most serious risk arises from hepatitis B but tuberculosis is still — one might almost say, traditionally — seen to be of serious concern and AIDS probably arouses more concern than all the others put together. In the future, hepatitis C is very likely to present a serious problem although experience with hepatitis B should help in developing a strategy to manage it.

Hepatitis B

This is a particular risk where patients are admitted from areas of the world in which the disease is endemic or in clinics where intravenous drug abusers are seen. However, as can be clearly seen from Table 5.1, there has been a steady decline in the number of cases in all categories of health service staff. In the four years 1985–1988, 139 health service staff were reported to have developed acute hepatitis of whom 31 contracted the disease abroad. Only one of these affected persons died and he was a general practitioner of 60 years of age who had worked among patients with a high prevalence of hepatitis B whilst visiting abroad. Only dentists as a group failed to show a decline in the incidence of the disease and this was due to a curious

TABLE 5.1

MEAN ANNUAL NUMBER OF REPORTED CASES AND MEAN ANNUAL INCIDENCE RATES/10^5 OF HEPATITIS B AMONGST HEALTH SERVICE STAFF*

Category of staff	1975–9		1980–4		1985–8	
	N	Rate	N	Rate	N	Rate
Surgeons	1.2	12	2.8	25	0	0
Physicians	5.4	12	5.2	11	1.0	2
Laboratory workers:						
medical	0.6	27	0.4	16	0	0
scientific	2.6	18	5.6	37	1.5	10
Nursing	26.2	7	19.0	4	9.8	2
Dentists	2.4	17	2.6	17	2.8	16
Staff in institutions for the mentally handicapped						
	8.6	31	10.4	27	4.0	10

*Data for England only. Based on S. Polakoff, Acute viral hepatitis B, *Communicable Disease Report*, 21 July, 1989

pattern in incidence which was higher in 1985 and 1986 than in the preceding ten years but was followed by a complete absence of cases in 1987 and 1988.

The reason for the decline in the incidence of hepatitis B undoubtedly owes a great deal to the general availability and the increasing uptake of the specific vaccine; it certainly is not due to increasing care in disposal or handling of instruments contaminated with blood judging from the rate of sharps injuries. All those at risk of the disease should be offered the vaccine but they should be warned that protection is not absolute and that it is certainly not a substitute for good and safe working practices. It is particularly important to emphasize that sharps must be disposed of safely and that failure to do so, particularly if it places another person at risk may lay the individual open to prosecution under the *Health and Safety at Work Act* or under the COSHH regulations.

The policy on vaccinations varies from one health district to another but it seems most sensible to restrict it to those who are readily at risk (see chapter 7). In addition to a policy on vaccination there must be a written policy relating to the taking and handling of blood and for the disposal of sharps. In the event of a sharps injury, the procedure to be followed must be clearly understood and adhered to.

Hepatitis C

Hepatitis C (previously known as one of the forms of non-A, non-B hepatitis) is spread in a manner similar to hepatitis B and is probably as prevalent in the community. It is certain to become of concern to occupational health departments and indeed, we have already two needlestick injuries involving a patient with hepatitis C. Since there is no vaccine and no specific immunoglobulin, treatment of these injuries must remain somewhat empirical. Serum should be saved to check antibody levels if the injured member of staff does develop jaundice and 75 mg of normal human immunoglobulin given. Doubtless a vaccine against hepatitis C will be developed as the extent of the problem becomes better known and specific immunoglobulin will also become available in time.

Tuberculosis

The increased risk of pathologists contracting tuberculosis was first recognized in this country in the late 1950s but the number of cases arising in health workers now is small; there were 16 new cases reported to the Health and Safety Executive as qualifying for disablement benefit between 1983 and 1986, for example. The principal risks in hospitals still arise from handling infected material or conducting post-mortem examinations on patients who have died from or with the disease. Patients who are known to have the disease are not a great risk since the initiation of effective treatment will prevent the airborne spread of the disease. Those who are admitted with a vague illness and only found to be suffering from tuberculosis after some while in hospital are more of a threat although even so, prolonged and close contact is necessary before there is a real likelihood of staff contracting the disease themselves. This has an effect on the follow-up procedure for contacts.

All health care staff who come regularly into contact with patients or who regularly enter patient areas, or who are likely to be exposed to potentially infectious materials should have their immune status tested. The Mantoux test is the standard against which all others are judged but the most frequently used test of immunity is the Heaf test and this is reliable provided care is taken in the performance of the test (see chapter 7). Those found to be negative in a Heaf or Mantoux test are given BCG. It should be noted that this is not the usual practice in North America and some European countries where the routine is to carry out annual skin tests and investigate those who convert from negative to positive. BCG is not normally given in those countries and health care professionals who come to work in this country will almost always have a negative Heaf test and invariably refuse to have BCG. This being the case, it has to be made clear that they should not undertake work which will place them at high risk of contracting tuberculosis and they should be asked to sign a statement to the effect that they have been offered and refused BCG vaccination; they should also be offered annual tuberculin testing. Other staff who refuse BCG must also be treated in the same way and their managers should be informed that they are at risk of contracting tuberculosis and that they (the manager) must take this into account when allocating duties.

The follow-up of staff who come into contact with a patient with tuberculosis seems often to cause much more concern and work than it need. The list of 'contacts' may well include those who have passed through the ward on their way to another part of the hospital or those staff who did not actually nurse or minister to the affected patient in any way whatsoever. Only those who have had close and frequent contact with the patient should be included on the list of 'contacts'. The list should be prepared by the control of infection officer working with the ward manager and the manager of any other department whose staff might also have had the necessary degree of contact. When complete, the list is forwarded to the occupational health department so that the immune status of those on the list can be checked in their records. Those who are not immune or for whom there are no records must be Heaf tested and given BCG if they are negative and remain negative after re-testing in six weeks. Chest X-rays are not required since they are not effective at picking up early signs of the disease. Having established the state of immunity, and given BCG to those who may require it, there is nothing further which need be done except to arrange a follow-up appointment in three months in order to make sure that none of those involved has developed symptoms. Naturally, all those who have been contacts must be told that they should report any untoward symptoms at any time and if any do, then the question of having a chest X-ray, or making a referral to a chest physician must be made on clinical grounds.

AIDS

The AIDS epidemic has engendered a considerable amount of anxiety amongst health care staff, much of which has arisen from ignorance. The occupational risk of contracting HIV arises in the same way as that of contracting the hepatitis B virus although it is by no means as great. Apart from sexual contact, infection can only occur following the inoculation of blood or other body fluids. This may occur through a needle-stick injury, during surgery or autopsy, or if blood or other materials are splashed onto the skin, eyes or mouth. The virus may also gain entry through cuts or grazes on the skin or through eczematous lesions. A considerable volume of blood is required to transmit the virus, probably at least 0.3–0.5 ml. The number of health care workers who are known to have sero-converted is small, and follow-up studies of those who have had an accident involving a patient known to be HIV-positive suggest that the risk of sero-converting is about 1 in 250 (0.5%). This is a low risk, but not negligible given the poor prognosis.

Those who are involved in an accident with a patient known or suspected to be HIV-positive must be counselled and a specimen of serum taken for storage. The antibody status of the patient should be determined if not already known but antibody testing on the injured member of staff should not be carried out as a routine but only after the issue has been thoroughly explored; counselling is best done only by those with experience and who understand the nature of the disease and the implications of sero-conversion. Many occupational health practitioners may feel that they have nothing to offer in this situation in which case they should establish a liaison with those who will undertake to counsel members of staff should it become necessary. If individuals do decide that they wish to have their serum tested then this should be done at an appropriate interval after the incident which would generally not be less than three months unless there are clinical indications for doing it sooner.

Whether or not those who have had accidents which put them at risk of exposure to HIV should be given AZT (Zidovudine) is open to question and there are few human data to help resolve this issue at present. To be effective it is generally agreed that the drug must be given as soon as possible after the accident, and preferably within two or three hours. The drug is given in a dose of 200 mg every four hours including a dose at night but it is not clear for how long; a minimum of six weeks has been suggested. The drug is toxic and side effects such as nausea and vomiting may discourage patients from continuing with it. The most serious side effect of the drug is marrow suppression leading to anaemia and neutropenia. A balance has therefore to be made between giving a toxic drug with no proven efficacy in these circumstances and the low risk of sero-converting and perhaps progressing to the full-blown clinical syndrome of AIDS; a balance between doing nothing and doing something. Practitioners may be able to resolve their indecision by asking themselves what their wishes would be under similar circumstances but in the end, the choice must be left with the patient if he or she is truly able to make an informed decision.

Other Infectious Diseases

Apart from tuberculosis, there are relatively few other bacterial infections which are a serious and actual occupational hazard for health care workers even though the potential for exposure is great. There is a risk of contracting *Salmonella* from excreting patients and this is perhaps the infection which is likely to result in most time lost from work. Intimate contact with patients with meningococcal meningitis may require prophylactic treatment with rifampicin and those who are found to be carrying haemolytic *Streptococci* or *methicillin* resistant *Staphylococci* should have appropriate antibiotic treatment although in the latter case this is done to protect the patient, rather than the member of staff. Some outbreaks of Legionnaire's disease have been reported in hospitals and health centres but the risks here are not peculiar to these environments.

Other viral infections which may spread from patients to staff, include respiratory syncitial virus, *Herpes simplex*, pharyngoconjunctival fever and epidemic kerato-conjunctivitis. Female members of staff may need advice and counselling about the risks of cytomegalovirus during pregnancy but there is no evidence for transmission from patients to staff and there is no difference in the prevalence of CMV antibodies and the acquisition of infection between women of the same age working with known CMV patients and those working in other areas. There is no call for routine serological screening of female hospital staff since there is no evidence that CMV is an occupational hazard.

Experimental Animals

Those who handle experimental animals have been known to contract exotic diseases from them including some of the viral haemorrhagic fevers and tuberculosis from primates. In some animal houses rabies is a hazard and staff must be vaccinated, preferably by the intra-muscular route. The real risk of infection from handling animals, however, is from being bitten with the subsequent development of secondary infection in the wound.

It is important to remember that those who handle experimental animals run a considerable risk of developing allergic reactions to the proteins which may be encountered in dander, urine or faeces. The prevalence of occupational asthma amongst animal handlers is considerable, in part depending on the type of animal present. All those who regularly work in the animal house must be under medical surveillance and any symptoms of wheeziness, persistent cough or tightness in the chest must be reported to the occupational physician. Those who already have asthma should not be permitted to work in an animal house and base-line lung function tests should be carried out on all new employees as soon as possible after they take up their post and repeated annually. Anyone who subsequently develops asthma must be thoroughly investigated to establish whether or not there is an occupational cause and efforts must be taken to reduce exposure. Sometimes it is possible to re-locate the individual but where this cannot be done protective equipment must be provided. The most useful is an air-stream helmet which must be worn at all times when the affected individual is in the animal house and not merely when he or she is actually handling animals since the allergens may be present throughout the area in sufficient quantity to evoke an allergic response.

Genetic Manipulation

The early work on genetic manipulation was accompanied by some exaggerated fears about the possibility of the release into the environment of 'super-bugs'. Wiser counsels have now prevailed and a much more level headed approach is being taken to these experiments. All work involving genetic manipulation, however, must be reported to the Health and Safety Executive and a safety committee must be established to advise and supervise it. The occupational physician acts as medical adviser to the committee and althouth medical examinations are not compulsory it is recommended that all those who are engaged in genetic manipulation should be seen by the physician when they start and annually thereafter; on the first visit blood and serum should be taken and saved for later investigation in the event of the member of staff contracting an unusual febrile illness. The first visit should establish that there are no contra-indications to the member of staff engaging in this kind of work; contra-indications are few but it would clearly be unwise to allow an individual whose immune system was compromised to take it up. At subsequent visits, enquiries should be made about general health and any episodes of unusual infectious illness which should in any case be reported to the occupational physician when they occur.

CHEMICAL HAZARDS

Every hospital contains within its walls many hundreds of chemicals, mostly in pathology laboratories. If used safely and in accordance with proper codes of practice they should present little risk to those who work with them. The trend, certainly in chemical pathology laboratories, has been towards increased automation and the development of micro-methods which greatly reduce the volume of reagents to be used. In histology laboratories the use of solvents in tissue preparation may be unpleasant if not actually dangerous if the general or local ventilation is inadequate. In the past the use of benzene as a clearing agent for tissue sections had very little to commend it from the point of view of health and safety and it should now have been replaced with xylene; we have found benzene still in use in at least one famous London teaching hospital and stocks of this solvent held by others.

The chemicals which are currently considered to be of priority, at least so far as the COSHH regulations are concerned, are formaldehyde, glutaraldehyde, ethylene oxide, xylene, toluene and white spirit, anaesthetic gases, cytotoxic drugs and mercury. These will be considered in more detail.

Formaldehyde

Formaldehyde is well known as a fixative and preservative and all those who have undergone a medical training will recall the pungent smell of formalin in the dissecting room. It is a highly irritant compound and it may cause conjunctivitis with lacrimation, rhinitis, laryngitis and pharyngitis. Exposure to high concentrations is usually abruptly curtailed by the development of intense irritation of the eyes and upper respiratory tract. Effects which may occur with sub-irritant exposures include the development of contact dermatitis and asthma. The symptoms in asthma seem to be due both to hypersensitivity reactions and sometimes to a direct irritant effect. There is no convincing evidence to show that formaldehyde is a human carcinogen altogether tumours have been induced in experimental animals.

All those who are exposed to formaldehyde should have to be placed under periodic medical surveillance. Where exposure is thought to be substantial, then environmental monitoring may be considered in order to ensure that concentrations do not exceed the control limit of 2 ppm $(2.5 \, \text{mg/m}^3)$. In the body, formaldehyde is converted to formic acid and measurement of urinary concentrations may be considered as a method of control although it should be noted that there are no generally accepted biological standards.

Health surveillance should aim to elicit evidence of sensitization either of the skin or the lungs. Examination of the skin and respiratory system is hardly to be avoided although little is likely to be found in the absence of symptoms; similarly, it would be difficult to resist carrying out lung function tests even though they are unlikely to reveal anything which a good history or a clinical examination will not. The situation is clearly different in a member of staff who has symptoms which can be related to exposure. If occupational asthma is suspected then the patient should be asked to carry out two hourly peak flow measurements following exposure, using a mini peak flow meter. If the results of this are suggestive, then patch testing or provocation testing may be necessary to confirm the diagnosis but these must be undertaken only by those with the necessary expertise.

Glutaraldehyde

This compound is widely used in hospitals and clinics as a sterilizing agent for which purpose it is used in an activated form; activation is achieved by adding sodium bicarbonate to it to raise the pH above 7.5. It has particular application for the sterilization of endoscopes and for this purpose it is found in gastro-intestinal units, theatres, radiography departments and chest clinics but it is also to be found in many other departments throughout the hospital where it is used to wipe down fume cupboards, containment cabinets or other surfaces. Its efficacy as a sterilizing agent is not in doubt and its increasing use has tended to follow the increase in the number of patients with AIDS since it seems to have gained the reputation of being the only agent completely to kill the virus.

Glutaraldehyde is an extremely irritant compound as one would anticipate from its chemical nature and it can cause all the symptoms which follow from exposure to formaldehyde. It is a known sensitizer and may induce both dermatitis and asthma. There is no adequate means of biological monitoring; it is likely to be metabolized to glutaric acid (by analogy with formaldehyde) which would then enter other metabolic routes leading to α-keto glutaric acid and the tricarboxylic acid cycle or to glutamate and amino acid synthesis. The compound has an acrid smell and this and its irritant effect on the eyes and upper respiratory tract will tend to limit exposure where this is possible. All too often, however, the places in which it is used are not suitably equipped with local or general ventilation and exposure during clinical procedures or during the preparation of instruments is inevitable. Enclosed endoscope washers and sterilizers are on the market but suffer from a serious design fault in that the activated glutaraldehyde has to be changed manually and this may result in considerable exposure. Where there is a strong smell of glutaraldehyde it is likely that the exposure limit (of 0.2 ppm, $0.7 \, mg/m^3$) is being exceeded. Methods currently used to measure airborne concentrations actually measure the total aldehyde content and so when interpreting the results it is necessary to know whether glutaraldehyde is present on its own or in combination with others aldehydes (generally formaldehyde). Health surveillance of staff exposed to glutaraldehyde should be undertaken as for formaldehyde.

Ethylene oxide

Ethylene oxide is a sterilizing or fumigating agent which is particularly useful for treating materials that cannot stand heat or moisture. The main concern about its use is that it may be carcinogenic. This is a realistic concern since not only does the parent compound have an active epoxide group within its molecule but one of its break-down products, 2–chloroacetaldehyde (which it shares in common with vinyl chloride) gives positive results in the Ames' test. Mutagenic and reproductive effects have been demonstrated in experimental animals and early epidemiological studies in those exposed at work suggested that there might be an excess risk of leukaemia but several more recent studies have failed to confirm this observation.

The acute effects of exposure to ethlyene oxide include irritation of the eyes and upper respiratory tract and prolonged exposure has been incriminated as a cause of various neurological effects including incoordination, memory loss and delayed nerve conduction. Control of exposure requires engineering rather than medical controls and factors such as ensuring a post sterilization air purge and adequate aeration of the articles which have been sterilized to reduce the amount of ethylene oxide liberated when the sterilizers are unpacked are all important. Personal dosimeters are available but there is no generally acceptable method of biological monitoring and regular health surveillance is unlikely to be helpful. Ethylene oxide is subject to a control limit of 5 ppm $(10 \, mg/m^3)$.

Anaesthetic Gases

The original concern about anaesthetic gases stemmed from their physical properties particularly the dangers from fire and explosion. The introduction of halogenated gases, which are much less flammable or prone to explosion has allayed these anxieties and in the past two or three decades attention has been given to the possible risks to the health of those who may be occupationally exposed.

Most attention has been given to the reproductive effects following early reports that female anaesthetists were more likely to have spontaneous abortions or to give birth to children with congenital malformations than other women. In some studies the wives of male anaesthetists were also more than averagely likely to have a poor outcome of pregnancy. Since the early work in the late 60s and early 70s many other studies have been carried out and by no means all have confirmed the initial results. A number of the studies have had low response to the questionnaires used, there has been bias in reporting and control groups have often been inadequately defined and there has frequently been little or no information about the anaesthetics to which the subjects have been exposed or to the concentrations which have been present. Even allowing for all these deficiencies, however, the evidence does tend to support the view that women who are exposed to anaesthetic gases in theatres during pregnancy are more likely to have a spontaneous abortion than if they were not so exposed; there is probably not a significantly increased risk of them having children with malformations nor does it seem likely that their husband's exposure will affect the outcome.

There have been a small number of reports of operating theatre staff developing hepatitis following exposure to halothane but most cross-sectional studies have not shown any difference in liver function between theatre staff and others. Prolonged exposure to nitrous oxide has been associated with the development of a peripheral neuropathy which resembles that induced by lack of vitamin B_{12} and it has been shown experimentally that high concentrations of nitrous oxide may result in the oxidation of B_{12} causing inactivation of methionine synthetase which is required for normal synthesis of folic acid.

Since anaesthetics produce profound effects on the function of the CNS in those to whom they are administered it is natural that some attention should have been given to their effects on those who administer them. As might be expected, performance in psychometric tests (such as simple reaction time) are dose dependent and become apparent only at relatively high concentrations; there is little evidence that trace amounts cause a decrement in perfomance in psychometric tests.

All modern theatres now have scavenging systems and adequate general ventilation so that concentrations of waste gases in the atmosphere are not a hazard to staff. In some recovery rooms, however, particularly if they are small and poorly ventilated, concentrations may be substantial and so may they be in some dental and other out-patient clinics.

If the occupational health department is satisfied that concentrations within theatres, recovery rooms and clinics are low, then there is no reason why pregnant women should not continue to work in them. Some women will not accept any reassurance, however, and under these circumstances it is prudent and caring to arrange for them to work in another part of the hospital during their pregnancy although it should be made clear that the reason for the move is not that it is the work is considered harmful *per se* but to allay fears and remove anxiety. Clearly if conditions are such that exposure may be substantial, this is enough justification for recommending a change of location.

It has been suggested that exposure to halothane should be monitored by measuring the concentration of trifluoroacetic acid in the blood and/or urine at the end of the working week and tentative values for the maximum permissible concentrations in each have been given as 0.25 mg/dl and 10 mg/g creatinine respectively. The concentration of nitrous oxide in the urine correlates well with atmospheric concentrations and this offers a potential means of monitoring exposure to this gas. However, simple passive samplers are available to monitor exposure and this is probably the method of controlling exposure which will find favour with those actually at work.

Cytotoxic Drugs

These drugs are designed to interfere with cell replication and it comes as no surprise that they are both carcinogenic and fetotoxic. Under the circumstances in which they are used, these risks are far outweighed by the benefits which they confer on the patients to whom they are administered. That they may also pose risks to those who prepare or give them, however, has been considered only relatively recently. Nurses who handle cytotoxics have been found to excrete high concentrations of thioethers (which are non-specific metabolites) in the urine and it has also been shown that their urine may be mutagenic. In one study in which we were involved, the thioether concentration fell significantly after the nurses started to wear protective clothing when they prepared cytotoxics on the ward.

The long-term effects of absorbing small amounts of these drugs is not known but the perceived risks have been sufficient to lead to the introduction of much safer ways of handling them. In many hospitals it is now the practice to make up cytotoxics in the pharmacy using a laminar flow cabinet. The drugs are then sent to the wards or clinics ready for administration. Where they have to be prepared on the wards then staff routinely wear protective clothing which will guard against skin or eye contact and the inhalation of droplets; gloves made of PVC should be worn rather than latex since the former confer a greater degree of protection. All hospitals or clinics where cytotoxics are used should elaborate a code of practice which governs their preparation and administration and which details the procedure to be followed in case of accidents. There is an increasing trend in some specialties towards the administration of cytotoxics at home and this is an area which may well be overlooked when devising a code of practice; it is also much more difficult to monitor and occupational health departments must be careful that they do not neglect staff who work in the community who may face greater risks than those working in the more well regulated hospital environment.

There is not much which can be done in the way of health surveillance or biological monitoring although thioether estimation has been mooted as a means of control; urinary platinum concentrations may be used to monitor exposure to platinum based drugs. In our present state of knowledge neither has much to commend it as a routine procedure. It is important, however, to keep a register of staff who regularly handle cytotoxics if only to be able to answer queries which may arise in the future. Only someone who felt very secure would agree to pregnant women handling cytotoxics, particularly in the early stages of pregnancy.

Mercury

Mercury is still used to prepare dental amalgam although it is being superseded by newer materials. A substantial number of those who handle mercury do not seem to be aware that it volatalizes at room temperature, that the vapour is avidly absorbed through the lungs and that absorption can occur through the intact skin. Having said all that, however, the risks to dentists and dental technicians should be relatively low. Mercury is also found in clinical areas in the ubiquitous thermometers and sphygmomanometers — pandemonium usually follows the breaking of one or the other if the mercury spills onto the floor. Occasionally a patient bites the end off a thermometer and may swallow a small amount of mercury; no harm can come of this since metallic mercury is not absorbed from the gut. The response to spillage in a ward or clinic is not to evacuate the area since there is no possibility of any adverse acute effects but to clean it up with dustpan and brush aided by some adsorbent material; there are now a number of so-called mercury kits on the market which will deal adequately with spillages. It is sensible to have a small supply of these in the occupational health department and for this fact to be widely enough known that use can be made of them when necessary.

In the days when hospitals had instrument curators, mercury

poisoning was not a common hazard.

The serious consequences of inorganic mercury poisoning are its effects on the central nervous system and on the kidney. These cannot be expected to occur in hospital staff nowadays. There is some evidence that relatively low concentrations may be associated with subtle behavioural effects which can be picked up with appropriate psychometric tests but even these are unlikely to be found in the groups we are dealing with.

The key to controlling mercury exposure is to carry out environmental monitoring which can be done quickly and easily with a mercury 'sniffer'. This is a costly piece of equipment but it can be used by any of the nursing or medical staff in the department and it will give a direct read-out. The eight hour time-weighted exposure limit for mercury is $0.5 \, \text{mg/m}^3$ and in our experience the concentrations within most dental clinics is an order of magnitude lower than this. Only if this limit were approached or exceeded would it be necessary to consider biological monitoring and urinary mercury levels provide the most convenient method.

Solvents

Any inventory of hospital laboratories will be found to contain a large number of solvents but relatively few in any bulk. The exception is xylene which is used in quantity in histology laboratories for de-waxing slides. Xylene shares a number of properties in common with other volatile organic compounds; in excessive concentrations it may cause acute symptoms such as headaches and dizziness and, if exposure were exceptional, it would lead to unconsciousness. It need scarcely be mentioned that this will not occur under the conditions of normal use in a laboratory.

Toluene is not much used in laboratories but care must be taken wherever it is used since it is liable to abuse, unlike xylene which has a rather repellant smell. Toluene is hallucinogenic and there is increasing evidence to show that those who abuse it for long periods may develop severe and permanent brain damage which can give rise to cerebellar ataxia or to dementia. There is some slight evidence that prolonged, heavy occupational exposure may induce symptoms of lassitude, poor concentration and changes in affect in a few individuals. None has been reported in health care workers and it is unlikely that laboratory use represents a real hazard to health although many find the smell of xylene offensive. Atmospheric monitoring is easily carried out with detector tubes which will indicate whether or not a full scale hygiene survey is necessary and it is important that the ventilation in laboratories is adequate to remove what vapour there is in the atmosphere. There is no useful form of medical surveillance although biological monitoring can be undertaken by measuring the concentration of methyl-hippuric acid or hippuric acid in the urine when there is exposure to xylene or to toluene respectively; levels should not exceed 1.5 g/g creatinine in the first case or 2.5 g/g creatinine in the second.

The other solvent which is likely to be encountered in quantity in the hospital setting is white spirit which is used in oil based paints. White spirit is a mixture of aromatic and aliphatic hydrocarbons including some which are irritant; these account for the symptoms which may be experienced when painting in small, badly ventilated rooms. There has been some concern that prolonged, heavy exposure was associated with an increased risk of presenile dementia but work in this country has been unable to establish any such connection. Painters may be heavily exposed in some circumstances and some will be able to recount episodes of vertigo or unconsciousness; prompt and complete recovery following removal from exposure is the rule.

Oil based paints are used less often than in the past and if this trend continues then levels of exposure will also diminish. In parts of the hospital where the walls are frequently washed down, however, oil-based paints must continue in use since water-based substitutes would not last long. Because of the pattern of work, exposure tends to be intermittant and it would be unusual to find hospital painters whose eight hour time-weighted average exposure exceeded the limit of 100 ppm ($575 \, mg/m^3$), despite some occasional excursions above this level. Personal exposure can be checked using passive samplers but there is no means of biological monitoring. If a painter consults the occupational health department it is much more likely to be on account of dermatitis than any symptoms referable to the CNS and they should be given advice about the inadvisability of using paint solvents as hand cleansers.

In addition to white spirit, painters may be exposed to methylene chloride which is a constituent of some strippers. This is an interesting solvent in that it is metabolised to carbon monoxide which immediately binds to haemoglobin to form carboxyhaemoglobin; elevated levels of COHb may thus be found in those working with methylene chloride. Because of this at one time it was thought that exposure to methlyene chloride might result in an increased morbidity from cardio- or cerebro-vascular disease. There is no convincing epidemiological evidence to support this view, however. The use of paint strippers based on methylene chloride is on the decline but, as with most other solvents, personal exposure can be monitored relatively simply. It should be noted that methylene chloride is subject to a control limit of 100 ppm (350 mg/m^3) and so where it is used, the conditions of use must be carefully assessed. Routine measurement of COHb levels is likely to prove unhelpful and will almost certainly reflect smoking habits more faithfully than exposure to methylene chloride.

Asbestos

Asbestos is almost always found in hospitals where pipes are lagged. It is generally confined to areas which are not frequently entered and is not a hazard unless the lagging is damaged and fibres are able to escape into the atmosphere. During rebuilding or extensions, pipes lagged with asbestos are often encountered and a state verging on panic has been known to ensue. When dealing with anxieties about asbestos, occupational health personnel must emphasize that asbestosis and lung cancer occur only with prolonged and heavy exposure and that this will not occur in maintenance work in hospitals. The same is probably true for the development of pleural mesothelioma although there are some cases in the literature which do seem to have resulted from slight exposure to blue asbestos. Where signs or symptoms of asbestos related disease do occur in hospital workers it is most important to obtain a clear history of exposure both during employment in the health service and at other times. In one case in which we were involved, a hospital maintenance engineer developed a blood stained pleural effusion and it was claimed that he had been exposed to blue asbestos during his early years in the hospital service. However, there was no record of blue asbestos having been used at the hospital and close questioning revealed that prior to entering the health service, he had worked for a number of years for a company where exposure to crocidolite had been substantial.

Where possible asbestos lagging should be repaired to prevent escape of fibres but in many cases there is no alternative but to remove it completely. Removal must be carried out by a competent and experienced firm adhering closely to the regulations and with constant monitoring by a hygienist. It is unfortunate that many of those who have worked in the areas where asbestos is removed become alarmed when they see the massive precautions which are taken to prevent exposure during the removal. Some may also have read or been advised that ill-effects can follow exposure to a single fibre. Where this happens, then the occupational health department must give proper and reasonable advice to all those who have been exposed, or think they have been exposed, either singly or in a group. This may not completely allay the fears of the people concerned and there may be a demand for a medical examination. If this is what it takes, then it should be undertaken, and a detailed occupational history taken at the same time in order to be able to quantify the risk to each individual. Where it is slight, and where there is no clinical indication, chest X-rays should not be taken. Where individuals have a history of significant past exposure, a chest X-ray is justified but it must be read by someone with experience in the field and it should be classified according to the ILO classification. Having completed a medical examination, repeated re-assurances should be given to those who are found to be normal and no further action should be taken. Any requests for routine screening should be resisted since to set up a system of annual surveillance will seem at odds with any advice that exposures are and have been negligible and that ill-effects will not occur.

ENVIRONMENTAL MONITORING

It is hardly likely that there will ever be a call for large scale programmes of environmental monitoring in clinic or hospital premises but nevertheless, occupational health departments should provide themselves with the means for carrying out simple measurements, particularly in relation to COSHH assessments. We recommend that all departments have equipment with which they can carry out spot measurements of atmospheric concentrations of commonly encountered chemicals such as xylene and formaldehyde; a Dräger pump and the appropriate tubes would suffice perfectly well for this purpose. A mercury 'sniffer' may be useful in large departments which have responsibility for dental clinics both within the hospital and in the community. These machines tend to be expensive and their need should be properly assessed before one is bought; on the other hand, the arrival of the COSHH regulations has focused the minds of many dentists on their exposure to mercury and we have been able to carry out a number of surveys for private dentists for a fee which has helped to offset our original investment.

Those who use these pieces of equipment must be well trained so that the results are reliable. When using Dräger tubes for different compounds, for example, the technique may vary considerably and it is important that the manufacturer's instructions are faithfully adhered to if the results are to be valid.

Sampling strategies must be given some thought; for example, readings should be taken at a time when exposure is likely to be greatest; measurements should be taken close to those most directly exposed but also in other parts of the areas in order to get some idea of 'background' concentrations; it may be necessary to take measurements both with and without local (or general) ventilation systems at work so that their efficacy can be established. It is important that those who conduct the survey understand that inappropriate measurements are likely to be worse than no measurements at all. Finally it should be obvious that those who take the instruments into the field must be able to interpret the results to members of staff in the area being investigated or have quick and ready access to someone who can.

The results of simple monitoring can often allay anxieties about over-exposure but they can also be used to indicate where a more detailed hygiene survey may be required. Other forms of environmental monitoring are discussed in chapter 6.

Physical hazards

Physical hazards likely to be encountered in the health care setting include ionizing radiation, lasers and ultrasound; in addition there are a wide variety of ergonomic hazards which arise from the physical structure within which staff have to work.

IONIZING RADIATION

This is the oldest and the best understood of the physical hazards which are present in hospitals and clinics. Sources of ionizing radiation include diagnostic radiography, radio-isotopes used in diagnosis or treatment and sealed sources used therapeutically in the treatment of malignant disease.

The effects of radiation are generally considered under two heads, stochastic and non-stochastic, or random and non-random. Non-stochastic events occur only after a minimum dose of radiation has been received and thereafter an increase in dose is associated with an increase in the severity of effects and in the number of cells which may be transformed by the radiation. The effects are predictable and to a large extent, the effects in an individual can be accurately anticipated from a knowledge of the dose received. Examples of non-stochastic effects are skin erythema and ulceration.

By contrast, stochastic effects take place even with very low doses of radiation although the number of cells which may transform increases with increasing dose. However, the effects are chance phenomena which cannot be accurately predicted in an individual but can only be defined in terms of probabilities which have been derived from studies of large populations. The probability of an adverse effect taking place increases with increasing dose but the effect is the same, no matter what the dose. For example, the probability of contracting leukaemia following exposure to radiation increases the higher the dose but once contracted the effect is the same, whatever the dose level; for example, if leukaemia follows exposure, there is nothing about the disease which will then depend upon the dose which initiated it and its natural history and its outcome will be same for all initiating doses.

The main stochastic effect of radiation, and the one which naturally causes greatest concern, is the production of tumours of, for example, the breast, lung, thyroid or blood.

It follows that if the threshold for non-stochastic effects is never exceeded then no harmful effects will be noted in the workforce. To avoid stochastic effects, on the other hand, all that can be done is to keep the dose as low as possible in order to minimize the probability of such effects occurring.

Levels of exposure in health care settings are generally low but concern is usually expressed about the possibility of cancer production, of the risk of incurring genetic damage which may be passed on as an inherited disease and the risk of malformation or cancer caused by irradiation of the fetus. The magnitude of the risk varies from organ to organ as indicated in Table 6.1.

At present workers aged over 18 years of age are permitted an annual exposure of 50 mSv and trainees under the age of 18 a limit of 15 mSv. These doses are based on experience which has been gained from populations exposed to high levels of radiation such as the survivors of the atomic bomb explosions at Hiroshima and Nagasaki and of groups of patients who were treated with high doses of radiation in the past. Current thinking,

TABLE 6.1

RISK FACTORS FOR VARIOUS ORGANS

Organ or tissue	Risk/mSv/10^6	Outcome
Gonads	4	Serious hereditary defects
Breast	2.5	Breast cancer
Lung	2	Lung cancer
Bone marrow	2	Leukaemia
Thryoid	0.5	Thyroid cancer
Other tissues	5	Cancer

however, is that it would be prudent to keep the average dose to 15 mSv a year, where the average is calculated over five or ten years and if this becomes accepted and outlined in legislation, as seems likely to be the case, then some changes in work practices will almost certainly have to be made.

RADIATION PROTECTION

There are a number of pieces of legislation which govern the use and control of ionizing radiation in hospitals including the *Ionizing Radiation Regulations* 1985, the *Radioactive Substances Act* 1960, the *Medicine (Administration of Radioactive Substances) Regulations* 1978 and the *Ionizing Radiation (Protection of Persons Undergoing Medical Examination and Treatment) Regulations* 1988. The input of the occupational health department in the implementation of this legislation is slight although the occupational physician is usually part of the Radiation Protection Committee and may be the approved doctor if there are any classified workers on site. Each hospital will employ a radiation protection adviser who is generally a physicist with appropriate treatment and this individual has the responsibility of advising on all aspects of radiological safety.

All personnel who are likely to come into contact with ionizing radiation have some form of personal monitoring which is carried out by the use of film or thermoluminescent badges which must be worn on the torso. The badges are usually sent off every four weeks for reading and the result is recorded in a register. The minimum dose which can be detected by the badges is about 0.2 mSv so that where the dose is below this, a record of zero exposure is entered into the record. If a badge is not returned for processing then a nominal dose is entered into the register which will be 15 mSv divided by the number of reporting periods in the year.

Areas within the radiology department can be classified either as controlled or supervised; a controlled area is one in which the instantaneous dose rate exceeds 7.5 μSv/h, hence a worker in the area is likely to exceed 3/10 of the relevant dose limit. Access to such an area is restricted to classified workers or to those working to a written system of work through local rules. A supervised area is one in which a worker will receive a dose which will exceed 1/10 the relevant dose limit and access is restricted to authorised personnel. From this it follows that a classified worker is one who may possibly receive a dose which exceeds 3/10 of the relevant dose limit and such a worker is subject to stringent medical and dosimetric monitoring. It is extremely unlikely that any health care workers would require to be classified although they may be if the new dose limit of 15 mSv were to come into force.

If any worker is involved in an accident or any other incident which results in a high exposure, the radiation protection adviser must be informed and he or she will carry out an investigation to establish the cause of the accident and the dose received by the member of staff. If the dose exceeds 3/10 of the relevant dose limit, then the Health and Safety Executive (HSE) must be informed. Records pertaining to over-exposure must be kept for 50 years. If the dose received is high, then arrangements must be made to limit any further exposure so that the annual dose limit is not exceeded.

Precautions when Dealing with Radio-isotopes

Radio-isotopes can broadly be divided into two categories, sealed and unsealed. In sealed sources the radioactive materials are usually in powder or solid form and encapsulated in platinum, stainless steel or some other metal casings. There is very little danger of spreading radioactivity through contamination and the principal hazard is from the radiation emitted by the source. Examples of sealed sources are ^{137}Cs and ^{60}Co needles and tubes, ^{198}Au grains, ^{192}Ir wires and ^{90}Sr β–ray applicators. Most of these sources are used in radiotherapy and many are reusable with a working life of about ten years. They must therefore be stored in a safe room with sufficient shielding. These sources are generally of high activity and must not be handled directly with the fingers.

Unsealed sources come in liquid or colloid form and are radionuclides used for diagnosis, treatment or research. Examples include ^{99m}Tc, ^{131}I, ^{32}P, ^{51}Cr and ^{59}Fe. When handling unsealed sources a hazard may arise either from external irradiation or from internal irradiation if the substance enters the body. As they are unsealed, a further hazard may arise from contamination.

When handling sealed sources there are three cardinal rules

to be observed: shielding, speed and distance. Adequate shielding will reduce exposure and this is generally achieved by the use of lead bricks and lead glass windows. Operations involving sealed sources must be carried out with the greatest speed possible since the dose received is directly proportional to the time of exposure. Sources should be manipulated with long-handled tongs and never with the fingers since the dose falls off as the square of the distance from the source. All swabs, dressing and linens used in the insertion of an implant must be tested with a radiation monitor before they can be disposed of and the patient must also be monitored to ensure that no source has been left behind.

The same precautions apply to unsealed sources but extra care has to be taken to ensure that the environment does not become contaminated. The laboratories in which they are used should have smooth non-absorbent surfaces so that they can be cleaned down and decontaminated easily and staff should wear protective clothing and waterproof gloves. All sources should be placed on a drip tray in a fume cupboard so that in the event of spillage the spread of the source is confined to the tray. Standards of hygiene must be exemplary and food and drink must not be consumed in a laboratory in which radionuclides are used.

Patients who are administered a therapeutic dose of a radio-nuclide may present a hazard to the staff who are nursing them. Such patients should be nursed in a room on their own with integral toilet and washing facilities. The floor of the room should be covered with absorbent paper to contain the spread of contamination from urine, faeces or vomit. Disposable crockery and cutlery should be used and handled with caution. Nursing procedures which are not urgent should be postponed for as long as possible to allow for the maximum decay in radioactivity from the source. Protective gloves, gowns and overshoes should be worn by staff entering the room and when excreta, bed linen or other articles are handled. All articles should be monitored before they are removed from the room.

Health surveillance

The average dose which is received by hospital staff is well below the annual dose limit and there is no call for any other kind of health surveillance. Annual — or more frequent — blood counts have nothing whatever to commend them and have no part to play in the supervision of workers exposed to ionizing radiation.

Lasers

Lasers have been introduced into medical practice on a consider-able scale during the last decade or so and they find many applications. They are especially common in ophthalmology where they are used in photocoagulation of the retina in diabetes and macular disease and to perform capsulotomy after cataract implant surgery or iridiotomy in narrow angle glaucoma. Other applications include the treatment of cervical cancer, vocal cord and tongue surgery, the palliative relief of airway obstruction in lung cancer or oesophageal obstruction in cancer of the oesophagus or stomach, the removal of brain tumours, the coagulation of bleeding gastric ulcers and the removal of birthmarks. Different types of laser are used in these various applications as shown in Table 6.2.

The principal hazard from lasers is the damage which is caused by heat, particularly when the laser is focused and lasers are classified according to their power output (*see* Table 6.3); a comparison with the data in Table 6.2 shows that all medical lasers fall into class four. The two organs which may be directly affected by lasers are the eye and the skin although it is the case that most injuries occur as the result of electrical burns from the extremely high voltage equipment needed to generate laser light.

The eye   The eye may be affected by intrabeam exposure, that

TABLE 6.2

LASERS IN MEDICAL USE

Type	Power	Uses
CO_2	1–30 W	Gynaecology, ENT, ophthalmology
Nd-YAG	1–100 W	Gastroenterology, chest medicine, ophthalmology
He-Ne	1 mW	Aiming beam
Dye	0.1–0.5 W	Photodynamic therapy
Argon	1–50 W	Dermatology, ophthalmology
Excimer	0.5–5 W	Ophthalmology

TABLE 6.3

CLASSIFICATION OF LASERS

Class 1	Power not to exceed maximum permissible exposure (about $100\,J/m^2$). Intrabeam exposure safe.
Class 2	Power up to 1 mW. Visible lasers only.
Class 3	Power up to 500 mW. Non-specular reflection safe. Intrabeam exposure hazardous.
Class 4	Power in excess of 500 mW. Extended source viewing and intrabeam exposure both dangerous

is to say, the direct entry of the beam into the eye, and by reflections from a shiny or other surfaces. Reflection from a shiny surface (specular reflection) is potentially more harmful than that from a rough surface (extended source viewing) because the power of the beam is not attenuated.

If the laser beam is of a long infrared (IR) wavelength, the light is absorbed at the front of the eye and damage is sustained by the cornea. At shorter IR and visible wavelengths the light penetrates to the back of the eye and causes retinal damage.

The skin   Damage to the skin is more likely to occur than damage to the eye simply because the surface area exposed to the beam is so much greater. Accidental exposure may cause a painful burn but is of much less consequence in the long-term than damage to the eye.

Protection of Staff Exposed to Lasers

When operating lasers, great care must be taken to protect the skin and the eyes (and — it goes without saying — those of the patient also). Great care must also be taken to avoid fire risks. The skin is relatively easily protected by gowns and other clothing. To avoid the laser beam damaging the eye, operators must avoid looking into it and reflecting surfaces must be either removed from the area or covered. Operators must wear goggles and it is essential that these are of the correct thickness and colour. To reduce the output of a 10 W class four laser to a safe level of 1 mW, for example, the goggles need to be not only of the correct optical density but they must also be able to absorb light of the desired wavelength. Goggles should have orange lenses when blue-green argon light is used, blue lenses for red helium-argon light, green for IR wavelengths and clear lenses for UV light. When laser beams are used with endoscopes it is essential that the eyepiece is fitted with a filter of the correct colour.

It is illegal to use two different lasers in the same room since each set of operators will be using goggles which are inappropriate for the other's beam.

All medical lasers must be housed in rooms with opaque windows and a safety lock on the door which automatically turns off the laser should anyone enter unexpectedly. The laser itself must be interlocked so that if the safety casing is removed the beam is automatically turned off.

Health Surveillance

When lasers were first used there was a vogue for detailed and regular medical surveillance of those working with them. With more experience, however, it is evident that this is not necessary. Periodic eye examinations have little or no part to play in the control of those exposed to lasers since it is unlikely that minor macular lesions will be detected either by an ophthalmologist or the individual and it is impossible to differentiate between laser-induced lesions and those resulting from other conditions if more than a week has passed since the putative exposure. When significant retinal damage has occurred there is no treatment which can be offered to the individual who, in any event, will not need to be told that he or she has a damaged eye by an ophthalmologist. The exception to this is when there has been an accidental exposure, and then the individual involved should be examined by an ophthalmologist and a detailed investigation into the circumstances of the accident must be investigated. Many theatres keep a detailed register of all laser use and this practice has much to commend it.

Recently it has been shown that ophthalmologists who have used blue green argon lasers for extended periods have a change in colour contrast sensitivity. This loss appears at the end of a working session and recovers by the next day. What the significance (if any) of this effect is by no means clear and it would be premature to suggest that all those using blue lasers should have this function routinely tested.

Ultrasound

Many ultrasound techniques are used in medicine for both diagnostic and surgical purposes, but whereas the diagnostic uses are widespread and increasing, the surgical uses are still somewhat limited. In surgery, ultrasound is used either to increase or modify the effectiveness of a surgical instrument or it is used alone to effect some surgical action. The most common use of ultrasound in surgery is in the treatment of Meniére's disease and focused ultrasound beams have also been used to treat glaucoma. Ultrasound devices are also used to emulsify a cataract to facilitate its removal by aspiration. In dentistry, ultrasound devices are used for removing calculus and other deposits from teeth.

Tools driven by ultrasound have been used for many years now to disintegrate renal or gallstones. When treating renal stones the lithotripter is held to the shoulder rather like a rifle with the ultrasonic source to the operator's ear and the barrel, along which the ultrasonic beam is transmitted is introduced through a nephrostomy into the patient's kidney. When the lithotripter is in use, sound levels may exceed the permissible occupational limits.

Health Effects of Ultrasound

There is to date no firm evidence that any harm results from exposure to ultrasound. There appear to be no adverse effects on the fetus or on children who were exposed to ultrasound *in utero*. Nor has there been any evidence to suggest that those exposed to ultrasound in industry suffer any damage to their hearing; although a pilot study of urologists using ultrasonic lithotripter did show a small but significant temporary threshold shift of between 5 and 10 dB. This suggests that the equipment may need to be re-designed to limit noise emission and that those who use it may benefit from periodic audiometry. Some consideration should also be given to the provision of hearing protection to the operator and other theatre staff who may be in close proximity to the equipment.

Ergonomic Factors

There are three main areas in hospitals and clinics in which
ergonomic factors may contribute towards discomfort or ill
health, or at least to perceptions of ill health. These are during
patient lifting and handling, in offices where poorly designed
furniture is being used and during the use of visual display
terminals (VDTs).

Back pain is one of the most serious occupational hazards in
nursing and is almost always caused by lifting or handling
patients (*see also* chapter 11). It is often the case that nurses
have inadequate advice on lifting during or after their training
and few hospitals employ a physiotherapist specifically for this
task and to give remedial therapy to staff once they have suffered
a back injury. Much of the time lost from work due to back pain
could be avoided if the injured member of staff could have active
treatment and rehabilitation; where this is available, the rewards
are immediate and obvious.

In industry no-one would be expected to move weights in
excess of ten stone without proper lifting gear, but this is an
everyday occurence on any adult ward. Nurses may work in
pairs but there is often a disparity between their size and strength
so that one may end up doing a disproportionate amount of the
work on his or her own. The beds are invariably of such a height
that the lifting has to be carried out with the back bent or
rotated, or both. Lifting gear is almost never to be seen.

When discussing back pain with occupational health practitioners one almost always experiences a feeling of profound
frustration because there is so little which can be done to prevent
it from occurring, although the encouragement of positive fitness
has some value. Despite an immense amount of research and
experience into the causes of back pain in nurses, there has been
no move to provide beds of the right height, equipment with
which to lift heavy patients or adequate training. Nor is there
very much which can be done to select out those who may be
most at risk. There was once a view that very tall women should
not be recruited into nursing but this is now no longer thought
to be either beneficial or practicable. Ultrasonic measurement of
the diameter of the spinal canal has been advocated as a pre-
employment screening device in some industries where back
pain is a hazard on the assumption that those with a narrow

canal are more at risk. The evidence on which this suggestion is based, however, is not very secure and even if it were, it would not be at all practicable. Probably the only sensible step is to persuade applicants for training with a history of back pain that they should look for a less arduous career.

Back pain is by no means the sole prerogative of the nursing profession; many clerical, secretarial and portering staff also suffer, largely because of the poor quality of their office furniture and the lack of lifting aids. A survey of the average health service office is not an uplifting experience. The space is generally cramped, often badly lit and heated and the furniture is archaic. Most complaints of back pain can be traced to the incongruity between the height of the chair at which the individual sits and the desk at which they work. It is absolutely essential that office chairs can be adjusted up and down and preferable that the back rest can be moved backwards and forwards. The cost of providing decent chairs is not great and in these cost-conscious days can be justified in terms of increased production and savings in time off work.

Hospital offices, like others, should be well lit, well heated, well ventilated, and the humidity should not be allowed to fall too low. Noisy printers should be shielded or placed in another room and photocopiers which are frequently used should be in a dedicated, well ventilated room. Individual practitioners will know how well the office accommodation in their own establishments meets these basic requirements.

VDTs have sprung up in great profusion in hospitals in the last decade or so and despite the massive amount of research which has failed to demonstrate any harmful effects of their use, operators continue to view them with alarm. Probably the most consistent complaint is that the use of VDTs adversely affects vision; in fact, of course, their use merely brings to light a pre-existing problem which the operators cannot overcome because they sit at a fixed distance from the screen. It is probably useful to test mid-point vision in VDT operators *before* they start work so that those who have a defect can be forewarned and advised to obtain glasses. There is no virtue in any form of annual or other screening unless the employer has determined what is to be done when abnormalities are found. Work with VDTs has no adverse effects on the fetus but some operators do not find the reiteration of the latest research findings of any comfort whatsoever and where this proves to be the case, it is prudent to find them some other work if this is possible. It must be made clear, however, that the reason for recommending relocation is not to remove the operator from any harmful emanations from the VDT but to alleviate the stress generated by continuing in the present work.

MONITORING THE PHYSICAL ENVIRONMENT

No occupational health department within the health service needs to be able to carry out detailed surveys of the physical environment but, as in the case of the chemical environment, they should be able to undertake some simple measurements. Every department should be able to record the temperature and humidity in work places since aberrations in these frequently contribute to a feeling of discomfort if nothing more serious. Most hospitals are over-heated, relatively poorly ventilated, seldom have air conditioning and are usually too dry. Any combination of these may lead to staff complaining of dry eyes, dry mouth and a dry throat often with an irritating cough. If the atmosphere is too dry and the floor covered with carpets made from artificial fibres, then the staff may build up a considerable static electric charge which will discharge when they touch metal objects such as filing cabinets.

If this were not enough to contend with, lighting levels are often poor and it is unusual to find staff given desk lamps which they can adjust to suit themselves; it goes without saying that they can usually do nothing to modify the temperature or humidity themselves. Some staff may find themselves so out of sympathy with their surroundings and so frustrated that they are unable to control them, that they may manifest more serious, albeit non-specific symptoms such as headaches, malaise, musculo-skeletal aches and pains, chest pains and shortness of breath; in short, that constellation of symptoms which is often referred to as the sick building syndrome, although it is not the building which is sick but the people within it. Simple adjustments to humidity and lighting may often relieve the symptoms and recommendations based on simple environmental measurements tend to carry more weight with management than those based on observation alone. Where simple remedies fail, it may be necessary to consider a review of the ventilation system which, unless it is properly maintained, can all too easily get out of balance and become ineffective.

Similarly, although noise levels in hospitals are seldom of such a magnitude as to raise concern, printers and ventilation systems and old trolleys run on uncarpeted corridors can often cause a nuisance and it is surprising how therapeutic a noise level meter can be in such situations. The investment required for a simple instrument will almost certainly be amply rewarded.

CHAPTER 7

Protection from infection

Many infectious risks from exposure to patients and their body fluids can be significantly reduced or prevented by effective vaccination programmes. Few vaccines give absolute protection however, and good clinical practice is essential if maximum protection is to be afforded. The practical aspects of vaccination and follow-up procedures after exposure to infectious diseases are an important function of occupational health departments. There is an additional role requiring screening and monitoring of staff for some infectious conditions — carriers of haemolytic streptococcal and antibiotic resistant staphylococcal organisms for example — which while not necessarily causing clinical illness in the carrier, nevertheless may create a risk for patients.

Staff are at varying risk from infection because of local variations in incidence and prevalence of disease. Different policies for protecting staff may be recommended by local control of infection committees, especially where some methods of protection are costly and economies are being sought. Occupational health practitioners may therefore find themselves being asked to carry out policies which are inconsistent with those in other hospitals or communities. It is important that practical procedures are rationalized as far as possible and inconsistencies removed. It is necessary to be familiar with the issues not only of infection control but also with the medico-legal and health and safety legislation required for protecting staff from risk at work. It is these latter commitments which are at times forgotten or insufficiently recognized when infection control policies are drawn up. The occupational health practitioner must ensure that all factors are considered when policies are being initiated or revised.

TUBERCULOSIS

In many European countries the incidence and prevalence of pulmonary tuberculosis has continued to fall since the end of the nineteenth century. Immigration to Europe from parts of the world, especially Asia where rates remain high, has created local exceptions to this trend. This is particularly noticeable in urban industrialized areas where work is readily available and to which immigrants are attracted. The overall incidence of the disease in all health care workers in the UK is similar to that of the population as a whole (10 per 100 000). Some occupations however, have higher incidence rates — doctors and mortuary attendants for example — with rates of 59 and 108 per 100 000 respectively (1980–84).

Cases of pulmonary tuberculosis are not always diagnosed at the time a patient is admitted to hospital and staff may be unknowingly exposed before the diagnosis is made. It is essential that staff who have direct contact with patients or pathological materials should be given maximum protection. This will mean that many occupations in addition to doctors, nurses and laboratory workers will require screening and, if necessary, protection. Tuberculosis in the UK is a prescribed industrial disease for health care workers whose work exposes them to risk of infection.

Vaccine BCG

This is a live bacterial vaccine containing an attenuated form of human tubercle bacillus — bacillus Calmette-Guérin (BCG). It is prepared in a freeze-dried form and must be reconstituted at the time of using. Once made up the vaccine should be used within two hours. Before the vaccine is given it is essential to assess for existing immunity. BCG should not be given to anyone who already has immunity to tuberculosis. When BCG is given to an immune subject an accelerated immune response occurs in about 24 hours. This reaction is painful, reddened and tensely swollen. It usually breaks down into ulceration.

Assessment of immunity is carried out by tuberculin testing, details of which are given later in the chapter. Positive tuberculin reactors should *not* be given BCG. Those who are tuberculin negative and who have not had previous BCG should be protected.

Those who are tuberculin negative but who have a history of previous BCG, provided a satisfactory scar can be identified, should not be given further BCG. A scar can generally be accepted as satisfactory if it is four or more millimetres in diameter. A typical scar is usually easily identified, being circular, smooth and colourless, with a diameter of four to ten millimetres. If a previous BCG scar cannot confidently be identified in a tuberculin negative subject further vaccine must be given. It is sometimes, for example, difficult to be confident about an irregular BCG scar which is surrounded by multiple acne lesions.

The recommended site for giving the vaccine is at the insertion of the deltoid muscle on the left arm. The vaccine must be given strictly intradermally. The dose is 0.1 ml. This should be drawn into a tuberculin syringe and a $3/8''$ 25 G (0.5 × 10 mm) short bevelled needle used to give the injection. In order to give the injection accurately intradermally, it is important to have the arm at the correct angle and this can only be achieved if the hand is placed on the hip with the arm abducted from the body. If the site of the deltoid is exposed by a garment being pulled over the shoulder the arm is inevitably held close to the body, which makes it extremely difficult to give an accurate intradermal injection. A correctly given intradermal injection results in a tense white raised bleb and considerable resistance is felt when the fluid is being injected. If little resistance is felt when injecting and a diffuse swelling occurs as opposed to a tense white bleb, the needle is too deep.

The subject must always be advised of the normal reaction to the injection. A small papule develops at the site of the injection approximately seven days later. This gradually widens into a circular area up to ten millimetres in diameter with scaling, crusting and with occasional oozing. It is not necessary to protect the site from becoming wet during washing and bathing. Should any oozing occur, a dry plaster is recommended.

It is important that all BCG sites are inspected six weeks later to ensure that there has been a satisfactory result and that no adverse reaction has taken place. All reactions must be recorded by measuring the transverse diameter in millimetres. A scar of four millimetres or more is satisfactory. Minor ulceration at this time will usually heal if protected by a dry dressing. Large ulcers and abscesses represent abnormal reactions and should be referred to a chest physician and, if severe enough, reported to the Committee of the Safety of Medicines. As a rule, abscess formation inevitably means that the injection has been given too deeply. Severe ulceration can also result from too deep an injection and also when BCG has been given to tuberculin positive subjects in error or to those who have had previous BCG. The purplish–pinkish colour of the scar at six weeks usually fades during the next three to four months to a colourless scar. Immunity to tuberculosis develops six weeks after the initial injection provided a satisfactory reaction can be demonstrated.

When BCG vaccine has been given nearer to the acromio-clavicular joint there is an increased liability to keloid scar formation and when given over the acromio-clavicular joint at least 90% of all scars will become keloid.

Occasionally an accidental inoculation of a finger occurs from a needle which has been used to give BCG with the risk that a tuberculous abscess may form in the finger pulp. It is recommended that in these cases anti-tuberculous treatment should be considered to avoid severe abscesses.

Contraindications to BCG

The vaccine should not be given to subjects who have or are suffering from:

1. Corticosteroid or other immunosuppressive treatment, including radiotherapy
2. Lymphoma, leukaemia or tumours of the reticuloendothelial system, including Hodgkin's disease
3. Reduced immunity due to hypogammaglobulinaemia
4. AIDS
5. Positive reaction to tuberculoprotein
6. Malaise and pyrexia.

The vaccine should not be given into eczematous areas of skin. An interval of three weeks should exist between BCG and any other live vaccine regardless of which is given first. Further immunization should not be given in the same area for at least three months to reduce the possibility of regional lymphadenitis.

Pregnancy

No adverse effects on the developing fetus have been reported but it is wise to avoid giving BCG during pregnancy.

An alternative strategy to BCG

In the US and some European countries BCG is not given routinely to health care workers. As an alternative, staff are monitored for exposure to tuberculosis by annual tuberculin testing to identify those who convert to being tuberculin positive. Converters are regarded as being infected and are started on anti-tuberculous treatment. A potential disadvantage of this policy is that repeat tuberculin testing may boost a minimal tuberculin reaction into becoming a positive response. Considerable care and experience is needed to ensure that this booster phenomenon is not wrongly interpreted and that anti-tuberculous treatment is not given unnecessarily. Another objection in principle is that this policy treats rather than prevents disease.

Tuberculin testing

The essence of the test is the introduction of tuberculin protein into the skin and subsequent observation of the site for an indication of hypersensitivity to the injected protein. Tuberculin is derived from the tubercle bacillus. The original form contained the unrefined extracts of the whole bacteria and was called old tuberculin (OT). A more refined version — purified protein derivative (PPD) — is used today.

There are several methods for introducing tuberculin into the skin, the most common in the UK being the Mantoux, Heaf and Tine tests. Before undertaking tuberculin testing it is essential to be familiar with the various factors that can influence the accuracy of the test. In the absence of such knowledge, tuberculin testing can result in subjects being wrongly selected for BCG and avoidable adverse reactions to the vaccine occurring. Positive reactions to tuberculin protein may be suppressed by the following factors:

- glandular fever
- viral infections in general, including those of the upper respiratory tract

- live viral vaccines
- Hodgkin's disease
- sarcoidosis
- corticosteroid therapy
- immunosuppressing diseases, particularly HIV

Subjects whose responses are negative at a time when they may have an upper respiratory tract or other viral infection should be re-tested two to three weeks after clinical recovery before being given BCG. Tuberculin testing should not be carried out within three weeks of receiving a live viral vaccine. Immunization programmes should be arranged so that tuberculin testing is carried out before live viral vaccines are given.

The following factors may also affect the consistency of tuberculin testing or add to its variability:

1. Tester/reader variation. Even in the best controlled trials there can be a significant difference between the results of one tester and reader against another.
2. The time at which the test is read. For a given test the majority of subjects will be positive at a given time. Some however, may be positive at an earlier or later time and will be misinterpreted at the standard reading time. This can lead to BCG being given in error.
3. The site. Skin thickness and reactivity vary in different sites of the body. The test should therefore always be standardized at the recommended site, which is on the flexor surface of the left forearm, at the junction of the upper third with the lower two thirds.
4. Repeat testing at one site may alter the reactivity either by hypo- or hypersensitizing the skin. In such instances a changed response from subsequent testing may reflect local change in sensitivity only.
5. Tuberculin absorption. Tuberculin can be absorbed on to materials and once tuberculin has been drawn into a syringe it should be used within 30 minutes otherwise there may be a deterioration in the tuberculin.
6. Age and sex. There is a tendency for the tuberculin response to diminish with age and this may be more pronounced in females.

Strongly Positive Tuberculin Responses

In some subjects sensitivity to tuberculin protein may be sufficiently strong to result in ulceration at the test site. Do not therefore unnecessarily re-test such individuals when it is possible to obtain confirmation of a previous strong reaction.

Mantoux Test

This is the most accurate tuberculin test and the one against which other tests are compared. Three strengths of tuberculin are available, 1:10 000, 1:1000 and 1:100. When selecting subjects for BCG the dilution used must always be 1:1000 of the purified protein derivative (PPD). At the recommended site 0.1 ml of this solution is injected intradermally. A standard 1 ml tuberculin syringe should be used with a 3/8" 25 G (0.5 × 10 mm) short bevelled intradermal needle. Considerable practice is necessary to perfect the technique of intradermal injections. A correctly given intradermal injection results in a tense white raised bleb and considerable resistance is felt when the fluid is injected. If little resistance is felt when injecting and a diffuse swelling occurs as opposed to a tense white bleb, the needle is too deep.

The test should be read between 48 and 72 hours. The majority of positive reactions occur at 48 hours. It is important to appreciate however, that a test result which is nearly positive at 48 hours may, if examined at 72 hours, become positive. It is important not to give BCG where there is a nearly positive reading at 48 hours without checking again at 72 hours. This may be difficult when large groups are being dealt with at one time and are being fitted in to a set timetable.

Only induration and not erythema should be recorded. The transverse diameter of the induration should be measured in millimetres. Where a measurement falls between divisions on the scale the lower division should be recorded.

Interpretation

0–4 mm   = negative
5–14 mm = positive
15 mm + = strongly positive

Always record the actual measurement of the test result and not just its interpretation. Unless the measurement is recorded there is no accurate information available for comparison with future tests.

Heaf Test

This is probably one of the most commonly used tuberculin tests in the UK. The Heaf gun consists of an end-plate and six needles attached to a firing mechanism and handle. The six needles are fired through corresponding holes in the end-plate. There are two settings for the needles, 2 mm for adults and 1 mm for children. Always check this before using. Magnetic disposable metal heads for the Heaf gun have been shown to produce a high false negative rate and these are not recommended.

A much stronger concentration of tuberculin is used, 100 000 units per ml of PPD. This must never be confused with the much weaker strength used for the Mantoux test. Tuberculin is placed on the recommended site of the left forearm using a glass rod or a platinum loop to distribute the tuberculin over an area of skin approximating to the diameter of the plate on the Heaf gun. The end-plate of the Heaf gun is then placed firmly and flatly over the skin and the mechanism fired. The test is read between five and ten days, most commonly at seven. Before using a Heaf gun it is essential that the user personally observes the sterilization of the gun. This is achieved by dipping the plate and needles of the gun in 95% spirit (Industrial methylated spirit BP) and igniting this to burn off, holding the gun at an angle of approximately 45° with the plate uppermost. It is essential to allow adequate time — approximately ten minutes — for the gun to cool. This must be emphasized, as it is not uncommon for errors to occur with burning of the skin through failure to achieve adequate cooling. When several subjects are being tested at one session three Heaf guns are necessary so that the cooling time causes no delay. The test is read as a series of grades from 0–4.

Grade 0 represents no response;
Grade 1 represents discrete induration at four or more points of penetration of the needles;
Grade 2 the induration around each needle site begins to merge with the next one;
Grade 3 the centre of the reaction fills with induration;
Grade 4 vesiculation or ulceration of the reaction takes place.

Interpretation

Grades 0 and 1 = negative
Grade 2 = positive
Grades 3 and 4 = strongly positive

Always record the grade and not only its interpretation. This will enable accurate comparisons to be made with future tuberculin tests.

The Heaf gun requires regular maintenance, with thorough cleaning after being used at one session. The needles should be scrubbed with a stiff brush using a hot solution of soap or detergent. Rinsing should be done with distilled water. The needles must be checked to see whether they are becoming blunted or slipping in the retaining plate.

Tine Test

This is a disposable tuberculin test consisting of four metal tines coated in dried tuberculin in gum acacia. When the tuberculin coating is thin and uniformly applied to the tips of the tines, this test is an effective and accurate one. In the past, tuberculin coating has not always been adequate. It has been shown to be thickened and globulated and retracted from the tips of the metal tines. In those circumstances the test does not perform accurately because the tuberculin is pushed back along the tines rather than penetrating the skin. The test should be read between 48 and 72 hours.

Interpretation Induration of 2 mm or more at one or more puncture sites is equivalent to 5 mm of induration from a Mantoux 1:1000 test. Doubtful reactions should always be re-tested with the Mantoux method before giving BCG.

Follow-up After Exposure to a Tuberculous Patient

It is not unusual for cases of pulmonary tuberculosis to be diagnosed in patients admitted for general investigation. It may be a week or longer before the diagnosis is made. During this time staff will be exposed to potential infection. It is now recognized however, that the diagnosis of pulmonary tuberculosis does not necessarily entail a risk to staff. Only those patients for whom tubercle organisms are identified on direct smear tests are regarded as being infectious risks to others. In those circumstances in which staff do need following up, the occupational health department must obtain the names of all those who have been at risk and their records must then be checked. Those who are recorded as being tuberculin positive, or who have had a successful BCG, need not have any further follow-up. Those for whom no record is present must be invited to attend the department for tuberculin testing. Negative responders must be re-tested in six weeks' time. Those who remain negative should be offered BCG. Any who convert during the six weeks to being positive should be referred to a chest physician.

It is recommended that strong tuberculin reactors i.e. 15 mm or more to a Mantoux test or grades three and four of a Heaf test, should have a chest X-ray following exposure to an infectious case. Where it is considered advisable to follow up exposure to a case of tuberculosis with a chest X-ray, it is important not to do this too soon. Most radiologists consider that significant lesions in the lungs will not be identified much before six months following the time of infection. Strong tuberculin reactors from high risk ethnic groups should be referred to a chest physician for longer term follow-up, even if their chest X-ray is clear at this time.

The Role of Routine Chest Radiography

There is no justification for a purely routine chest X-ray. Staff who are recruited to work in hospitals and other health care institutions should have chest X-rays only for specific reasons. These are:

- a history of recurrent cough for three weeks or more;
- recurrent episodes of chest infection;
- social or ethnic backgrounds where there are high incidence and prevalence rates of tuberculosis;
- all positive tuberculin reactors who have not had BCG
- and only strong tuberculin reactors among those who have had BCG.

Regular chest X-rays during employment, even for those considered to be at higher risk, provided they are tuberculin positive or have had BCG, are not recommended. Studies have confirmed that the low incidence of tuberculosis in these groups no longer justifies routine radiography. It has also been shown that routine films are not very effective in detecting early pulmonary tuberculosis. A review of the role of routine chest X-rays in the National Health Service in England and Wales (1980–84) showed that among staff who had routine chest films and who developed pulmonary tuberculosis over 60% were not detected by the routine film. The condition was only revealed after the presentation of clinical symptoms.

It is important to emphasize that the significant chest symptoms already described will always justify chest radiography. Cooperation with personnel departments will be essential to ensure that the causes of staff sickness absence can be identified and those with chest problems followed up appropriately.

HEPATITIS B

Although the incidence of this blood-borne disease is much lower in the countries of Northern Europe compared with most African and Far Eastern countries, the condition nevertheless poses a potential hazard to all health care workers who are exposed to patients or their body fluids. Transmission of the virus does not readily occur through healthy intact skin. Risk circumstances occur from sharps injuries from contaminated needles, infected blood splashing on to grazed or cut skin, or skin which is unhealthy due to dermatitis or eczema. Droplets sprayed into the eyes or ingestion of infected fluid may also allow transmission of the virus.

If an occupation places an employee at an additional risk from infection, protection by vaccination should be given. Occupational health practitioners must take an objective assessment of risk to all staff for whom they have responsibility. In addition to doctors and nurses, most paramedical and ancillary workers will require protection. Laboratory staff and mortuary attendants are also groups which are particularly at risk. It should not be forgotten that non-medical groups such as porters and security staff may also be at risk when dealing with violent patients. Student nurses are particularly vulnerable in their first six months or so of training because of the greater incidence of sharps injuries sustained by them during this time. It is important also to remember medical students, who should be protected when they start their clinical studies and particularly when they go to Third World countries as part of an elective programme during their clinical work. Maintenance staff in hospitals are also liable to sharps injuries when clearing blocked outflows from basins which have been obstructed by accidentally discarded needles.

In general, any worker who has a risk of an exposure either from sharps injuries or from uncontrolled blood exposure — ambulance workers for example — should be vaccinated. Some working areas in hospitals will be particularly risk situations because of the higher carrier rate of the virus among the patients. Examples of these are drug dependency and sexually transmitted disease clinics, infectious disease wards and mental handicap institutions, especially where the latter have cases of Down's syndrome. Male cases of this condition are six times more likely to be carriers than female.

Epidemiological studies have shown differential rates of hepatitis B amongst health care workers. These are particularly notable in surgeons, laboratory workers and staff in mental handicap institutions where the annual incidence rates in the UK are 25, 37 and 27 per 100 000 respectively, compared with a rate of 3 to 4 per 100 000 for the general population.

Although vaccination gives a high degree of protection this must not be regarded as the sole means of protecting staff. Good clinical practice is essential and should always be followed. Clinical procedures which may expose staff to blood or body fluids should be undertaken wearing gloves, appropriate plastic aprons and, if necessary, eye protection. This latter precaution is often neglected where there is the possibility of droplet spray. This may be particularly true in some operative procedures, dental work and in post-mortem laboratories.

All forms of viral hepatitis are prescribed industrial diseases in health care workers in the UK where their work exposes them to a potential risk of infection.

Vaccine

There are two forms of hepatitis B vaccine, both of which are inactivated. The first, a plasma based vaccine, has been derived from human subjects who are antigen carriers due to previous infections from hepatitis. The latter development is a yeast-derived vaccine produced by genetic engineering. Both vaccines have been found to produce good immunity. Antibody production tends to occur less well in older subjects, particularly those over 40 and less so in males than in females. In the under 40 year old age groups production of protective antibodies occurs in up to 97% of subjects.

Before the vaccine is given it is not necessary to test for existing antibodies. Some subjects are reluctant to accept the vaccine because they believe that a pre-vaccination blood test will include testing for antigen and that a positive finding could affect their suitability to continue in their particular career. General education of staff at risk is important to reassure them that no blood testing will be done before the vaccine, either for antibody or antigen. This may increase the numbers, especially of doctors, who will be protected.

The normal course of vaccine consists of three injections each of 1 ml, given intramuscularly into the deltoid muscle. There is one month between the first and second injections and five months between the second and third. If the vaccine is given into fat, antibody formation is poor; the buttock should not therefore be used. Care should be taken to use a sufficiently long needle introduced at right angles to the skin surface to ensure that it enters the deltoid muscle and not the subcutaneous tissue. If there is insufficient time to complete the normal course a shortened version can be given with an interval of one month between each of the three injections. When the shortened course is used, a fourth injection should be given in a year's time.

It is generally recommended that post-vaccination antibody assessment should be carried out three months after the third injection. If antibody levels are unsatisfactory at this stage a fourth injection should be given and further checks carried out three months later. If antibody levels remain unsatisfactory at this time it is advisable to wait a whole year before giving a fresh primary course. If an individual permanently fails to develop antibodies, a change of occupation may be necessary, depending on the degree of risk.

Antibody levels over 10 i.u. per litre give a degree of protection. It is generally agreed that levels over 100 i.u. per litre will give protection for up to five years and that levels between 50 and 100 i.u. per litre for three years. Those with levels between 10 and 49 i.u. per litre may be protected for up to two years. Booster injections should be given at the appropriate time intervals. In the interests of economy hepatitis B vaccine has been used intradermally using 0.1 ml of the vaccine. Intradermal injections are not easy to do and this technique is not accurately carried out in routine field use. If the small volume of 0.1 ml is given too deeply, antibodies will not be produced. Another potential disadvantage is that the aluminium content in the yeast-derived vaccine may cause local reactions at the site of the injection. This should be avoided. The intradermal method of giving the vaccine is not recommended for general use.

Follow-up After Exposure to a Risk Incident

The most common accident is from a sharps injury from a used needle. Where it is practical the patient concerned should be checked for hepatitis B antigen. If this is negative no further action is needed. In the event of a positive finding the immunization state of the injured member of staff must be checked. Those who have been vaccinated and have had satisfactory antibodies demonstrated need only have a booster injection of 1 ml of the vaccine if they are beyond the period of cover provided by the antibodies demonstrated after their vaccination course. Staff who are at risk and who have not been protected by the vaccine should be given an injection of 500 mg of hepatitis B specific immunoglobulin preferably within 48 hours of the risk and no later than seven days, and at the same time started on the first injection of the vaccine. It is not necessary to give a second injection of the immunoglobulin when the vaccine is started at the same time. Immunoglobulin should always be given intramuscularly and into the buttock because of the large volume of the injection. Recipients should be kept for 20 minutes afterwards in case of any acute reaction to the injected protein.

Unknown Sources of Risk

It is not uncommon for a sharps injury to occur to a member of staff from a needle, the source of which cannot be traced or identified. If the needle has come from a clinical area where hepatitis B infection is likely — a drug dependency clinic for example — the follow-up should be based on the assumption that a risk has occurred. In other circumstances it is probably not justified to give specific immunoglobulin. It is recommended however, that a course of hepatitis B vaccine should be started at once. It has also been recommended that a sample of blood should be taken from these individuals and the serum stored for six months against the possibility of hepatitis B subsequently developing. This may well be worth doing if there is some doubt about the possibility of linking a subsequent infection with the risk incident. However, for health care workers hepatitis B is a prescribed disease and the association with occupation should always be accepted. Taking blood samples for serum storage may be an unnecessary procedure.

MENINGOCOCCAL MENINGITIS

This serious and at times fatal illness caused by the bacteria *Neisseria meningitidis* occurs as a rule in isolated and spasmodic outbreaks in which only a few individuals contract the disease. It is probable that natural immunity exists in over 80% of the population. The illness may take a rapid course in which a patient suffering only from general malaise, mild headache and pyrexia in the morning may, by the evening, have lapsed into unconsciousness. Most deaths occur within 24–48 hours of admission to hospital. A fatal case will cause considerable anxiety among those who have been treating the patient but spread to doctors and nurses is rare. The main risk is to those who may have rendered mouth to mouth resuscitation to the unconscious patient. The seriousness of the illness and the anxiety generated among staff however, require that all who have been closely involved in treating the patient should be followed up. This will probably involve only doctors and nurses. Transient contact, when for example a porter takes the patient on a trolley from an ambulance to the ward, is not a significant exposure.

Vaccination and Prophylaxis

There are three strains of the meningococcal organism: A, B and C. Vaccines have been developed against strains A and C but not as yet against B. The latter strain predominates in the UK and vaccination does not therefore play a significant part in protecting staff. In other parts of the world, especially in the Middle and Far East strains A and C prevail and the appropriate vaccines afford significant protection.

In the UK prophylactic antibiotic treatment with rifampicin 600 mg twice a day for two days gives protection. It should be given within 48 hours of exposure to a case. To cope with out-of-hours situations it is recommended that the occupational health department should arrange for the pharmacy to prepare individual courses of rifampicin. These should be kept where they are accessible 24 hours a day. The accident and emergency department may be the most appropriate place for this if agreement can be reached with the manager of that unit. The control of infection officer and control of infection nurse should be advised of the arrangement as they will usually have the immediate responsibility of ensuring staff safety when occupational health staff are not available.

AIDS

The human immunodeficiency virus (HIV) is found in nearly all body fluids but its presence in blood raises most concern for health care workers. The virus, in contrast to hepatitis B, is not readily transmitted from a patient to staff in accidents involving contaminated needles and scalpels. It does not survive outside body temperature for much longer than three to four hours, which reduces the risk from discarded needles. Regardless of the low infectivity of the HIV organism good clinical practices are essential and should be meticulously followed at all times. Whether or not the patient is suspected of being an HIV carrier, protective gloves, plastic aprons and eye protection must be worn whenever there is a risk of contamination by body fluids or blood. It is particularly important to avoid scratches or grazes being exposed to infected fluids. Sufferers from eczema or dermatitis of the hands, arms or face should not remain on clinical duties until such conditions have resolved.

Meticulous care must be taken to dispose of used needles into sharps boxes. The majority of sharps injuries to nurses however, occur not from wrongly discarded needles but from self-inflicted injuries shortly after administering an injection to a patient, when the nurse's attention may be distracted. In operating theatres routine safety procedures must be followed including the immersion of used scalpels in disinfecting fluids (hypochlorite 1% or glutaraldehyde 2%) before removing the blades. Repeated trauma to the fingers from suturing needles during deep abdominal or pelvic operations remains of concern to surgeons. It has been shown that wearing double surgical gloves reduces the incidence of penetrative needle injuries to the skin during operations. In some hospitals it has also been advocated that protective thimbles on the tips of the fingers will also reduce the same risk. For most surgeons however, neither of these precautions leaves sufficient dexterity for them to exercise their usual skills. Dental practitioners should routinely wear surgical gloves and normally find no difficulty in undertaking their work with these.

Follow-up after a risk incident

There are probably few more difficult situations to deal with than when a member of the nursing or medical staff receives a sharps injury or cut from a needle or scalpel blade recently used on an AIDS patient. Reassurance about the remoteness of the possibility of any infection occurring from such an incident is difficult when the injured person is aware that cases of infection in such circumstances have occurred to health care workers — albeit very few. Fortunately, studies of large numbers of sharps injuries in the US have shown that the risk is extremely low and probably only exists when a volume of blood in inoculated at the same time as the injury. Other circumstances in which transmission of the virus has occurred from the patient to staff have been in instances where infected blood has contaminated eczematous skin. Immediately following a sharps injury the injured site should be encouraged to bleed and be thoroughly washed with soap. If fluids splash into the eyes, they should be well irrigated with water. A considerable amount of counselling will almost certainly be necessary to reduce the inevitable anxiety, and there can be an additional problem in that the anxiety may extend to their partner.

One of the practical issues facing the occupational health practitioner is the question of testing the member of staff for HIV antibodies following the injury. Conversion to HIV positive does not usually occur before three months from the date of exposure and may take as long as 12–15 months. In discussing and counselling about the relative merits of testing this point must be emphasized at the outset. Once a decision has been made to test there will be a three months' wait before the first test is carried out unless there is a clinical reason to do so earlier. During this time frequent contact with the person concerned is important to ensure that undue anxiety is not developing. On balance, experience suggests that a member of staff in these circumstances is advised to have the antibody test because of the high probability that it will prove negative and full reassurance can be given. This is of especial importance for those who are married and who are contemplating having children. It remains however, a matter of judgement and experience how any given case is best handled.

The Use of Zidovudine in Prophylaxis

The antiviral agent zidovudine, azidothymidine (AZT) has been used in treating AIDS patients and there is evidence that it can be of benefit in prolonging their lives. Consideration has also been given to using it as a prophylaxis for health care workers after sharps injuries. If zidovudine is used, it should be started as soon as possible after the risk incident and no later than twelve hours afterwards. It should be used for at least six weeks and be given at four-hourly intervals throughout the 24 hours. There is uncertainty about the long-term side effects from zidovudine. Known toxicity effects of the drug include anaemia, neutropenia and leucopenia, fever, myalgia and enhancement of toxicity of some other drugs. It is an extremely finely balanced decision whether or not to recommend this prophylaxis with unknown long-term side effects when the risk against which it is proposed to use it is extremely low. The balance of opinion at present is that sharps injuries which do not involve a volume of blood being injected do not justify the use of zidovudine. If a volume of blood has been injected, it may be justified to recommend a course.

When effective and safer antiviral agents are developed, prophylactic treatment for staff after sharps injuries from HIV positive patients will become routine practice.

RUBELLA

It is essential that all personnel, whether male or female, who work in antenatal clinics should be immune to rubella. This will ensure that staff do not carry or transmit the rubella virus to susceptible patients. In practice it is not realistic to protect only antenatal staff. Antenatal patients may attend a wide range of hospital clinics during their pregnancy. It is therefore recommended that all staff who deal with patients should be tested for the presence of rubella antibodies and those who are negative should be given rubella vaccine. Medical students should not be forgotten and should be screened and protected if negative, by the time they start their clinical studies.

Vaccination

Rubella vaccine contains a live modified form of the rubella virus. There is a theoretical risk that those who have been immunized may pass the virus to susceptible patients. In practice this is not a risk and those who have been immunized need not be isolated from the patients. One injection of 0.5 ml of rubella vaccine subcutaneously gives protection. Following immunization mild symptoms of rubella may occur in a few subjects approximately ten days later. There may be a rubella type rash, enlargement of the occipital glands, pyrexia and joint pains. Occasionally an arthropathy may last several weeks and may be disabling. It is always wise to warn those who are given rubella vaccine of the possibility of these side effects.

RABIES

This condition is not endemic in Great Britain and therefore there is no routine need for hospital staff to be protected. There are however, a few laboratories and units in the UK where animals are placed in quarantine to eliminate the possibility of them being rabies carriers. Staff who work in these laboratories and infectious disease units associated with them should be protected with rabies vaccine.

Vaccine

This is an inactivated preparation. The recommended course consists of 1 ml given intramuscularly or deep subcutaneously and a further 1 ml repeated one month later. A booster injection of 1 ml may be given six to twelve months later. Because the vaccine is expensive it is sometimes given intradermally using only 0.1 ml. A check by one of the authors on the levels of antibodies of staff who had been given the vaccine by the intradermal method showed that in a third of subjects antibodies had not developed. It is therefore recommended that rabies vaccine is always given intramuscularly or deep subcutaneously and not by the intradermal method. It is of particular concern that staff who have received the vaccine intradermally and who subsequently go abroad into areas where rabies is endemic will do so in the belief that they are protected.

TETANUS

It is generally recommended that the entire population should be protected against tetanus. For the majority of health care workers tetanus is not a specific occupational risk. It is recommended however, that manual workers, particularly maintenance staff and people who work out-of-doors in hospital grounds, and laundry workers, should be protected.

Vaccination

The vaccine is prepared from tetanus toxoid adsorbed onto aluminium hydroxide. The primary course consists of three injections each of 0.5 ml given deep subcutaneously. There is an interval of six weeks between the first and second injections and six months between the second and third. Booster injections of 0.5 ml should be given at intervals of approximately ten years. Too frequent boosters are unnecessary and give rise to allergic reactions to the aluminium component of the vaccine. It is also unnecessary to give a second primary course however long an interval there may have been since the original one. In the past there has been a general tendency to over immunize with tetanus toxoid, resulting in reactions to the vaccine. When there is a history of a possible reaction to a previous injection of the tetanus toxoid an intradermal dose should not be given because of the risk of creating a severe reaction in the skin. When there is a history of a previous reaction it must be a clinical decision alone whether or not to give a further injection.

POLIOMYELITIS

It is recommended that all health care workers should be protected against this disease.

Vaccination

A live attenuated viral vaccine is most commonly used. The primary course consists of three doses given orally at intervals of four to six weeks. Each dose consists of three drops of vaccine which can be placed on a lump of sugar, in a spoon or directly into the mouth. A booster dose of three drops should be given every ten years if there is a general risk of exposure to the disease. In the event of an exposure to a known case of poliomyelitis a booster dose is recommended even if the primary course has been given less than ten years previously.

The general guidelines on the use of live viral vaccines apply to this vaccine. An additional point arises in that the vaccine contains a minute quantity of penicillin. This is therefore a theoretical reason why the vaccine should not be given to penicillin sensitive subjects. In practice, the minute quantity of penicillin in the vaccine is insufficient to constitute a contraindication when someone is at risk from the disease.

There is an inactivated poliomyelitis vaccine which may be considered for staff caring for severely immuno-suppressed patients. The course consists of three injections each of 0.5 ml given deep subcutaneously or intramuscularly at the same intervals as the oral vaccine.

Poliomyelitis used to be called 'infantile paralysis' suggesting that older age groups were not at risk. This is not in fact true and it is recommended that all age groups are immunized.

SMALLPOX

Following the successful World Health Organization's programme to eradicate smallpox, routine vaccination against this
disease is no longer necessary, either for the general population
or health care workers. There are however, a few specialized
laboratories throughout the World where cultures of the smallpox
virus are maintained. Laboratory staff involved in this work still
require therefore to be vaccinated against smallpox. In the event
of a generalized vaccinial reaction there is now no specific
immunoglobulin available and it is essential to adhere strictly to
the contraindication to vaccination. The presence of eczema, all
immunosuppressing diseases and the taking of systemic steroids
must preclude vaccination. It is also essential to warn those
vaccinated that they must avoid contact with infants and young
children with eczema because of the danger of transmitting the
vaccinial virus and causing generalized vaccina which may be
fatal.

ENTERIC INFECTIONS

Salmonella and shigella organisms are the most common cause
of food poisoning in hospitals. Salmonella infections may occur
from meat, especially poultry, which is already infected before
entering a hospital. Routine screening of catering staff by stool
testing is no longer recommended. Good personal hygiene of
kitchen staff and thorough cleaning of food preparation areas
and equipment is of major importance in preventing spread of
infection. All food handlers should however be seen in the
occupational health department and careful histories taken about
previous episodes of diarrhoea and enteritis. Where there is any
history suggesting a previous infection with a pathological
organism, stool testing should be undertaken and work should
not commence until a clear result is obtained.

All food handlers must be instructed about the importance of
reporting gastrointestinal symptoms and diarrhoea, especially
on returning from holidays abroad. They should go off work and
remain so until stool clearance is obtained. Nursing, medical and
all other staff who deal directly with patients should be aware
of the risk of transmitting enteric pathogens to susceptible

patients, especially children. They must be trained to report episodes of diarrhoea and go off duty whenever there is a risk to patients. Confirmation of a negative stool culture should be obtained before returning to work in these circumstances. It will be necessary at times to exercise careful judgement about the need to insist on staff remaining off duty and being stool tested. No-one likes having to produce stool specimens and if too zealous a regime is enforced staff will simply cease to report their symptoms. It is better to encourage symptoms being reported in order that case clustering can be observed and common sources of infection identified.

HAEMOLYTIC STREPTOCOCCAL INFECTIONS

Wound infection by haemolytic streptococcal organisms can cause serious problems in surgical units. The organism may be carried by staff who have throat infections. Occasionally it may be carried on skin lesions. Whenever there are cases of wound infection from streptococcal organisms throat swabs should be taken from staff to identify carriers. Throat infections may be clinically evident in most cases but some carriers may be symptomless. For adequate control of this infection in hospitals close cooperation between control of infection officers and nurses and occupational health units is essential.

The majority of haemolytic streptococcal organisms remain sensitive to penicillin and those which are resistant are usually sensitive to erythromycin.

STAPHYLOCOCCAL INFECTIONS

Carriers of this organism are often symtomless. In outbreaks of wound infection widespread searching for carriers amongst staff may be indicated. The organism may be carried in the nose and on the skin especially in the axillae and groins. Methicillin resistant *Staphylococcus aureus* (MRSA) cause major problems in hospitals. Whenever one of these organisms is identified as a cause of wound infection extremely careful screening of staff must be carried out. The policies of the local control of infection committee must be followed. These usually require swabs to be taken from the nose, axillae and groins of all staff connected with the outbreak.

HERPES SIMPLEX VIRUS

This organism causes vesicular lesions on or around the lips. Sufferers often have recurrent lesions because of the tendency of the virus to remain dormant after resolution of a clinical lesion. Staff in paediatric units are prone to infections because of the presence of the organism in sick children. Application of acyclovir 5% cream to the area concerned immediately symptoms develop will abort lesions in approximately 75% of cases. It must be applied five times a day for five days. The value of this antiviral preparation lies in early applications and tubes of the cream should be readily available for staff at risk.

CYTOMEGALOVIRUS

Approximately 1% of newborn babies are seropositive to this virus, and the percentage of positive subjects in the population increases with age. There is a possibility that the virus causes congenital malformations. In general however, it has little significance as a cause of serious illness and there is no clear cut clinical picture in those who become infected. Fatal disseminated illness may occur in immunosuppressed patients. Serological studies are difficult to interpret and do not enable susceptible or immune subjects to be identified accurately and for all practical purposes the cytomegalovirus does not have any occupational health significance for health care workers.

INFLUENZA

Routine immunization against influenza is not recommended for health care workers. It is recommended for those who suffer from the following chronic diseases: bronchitis, emphysema, bronchiectasis, ischaemic and valvular cardiac disease and nephritis.

Vaccine

This is an inactivated vaccine derived from the surface antigen of the influenza virus. One injection of 0.5 ml given deep subcutaneously or intramuscularly provides protection for five to six months. The vaccine is contraindicated in anyone sensitive to egg or chicken protein.

GENERAL COMMENTS ON VACCINES

The majority of vaccines are inactivated. Some however, contain live attenuated organisms, usually viruses. If it is necessary to give more than one live viral vaccine at the same time they should be given simultaneously and at sites in separate arms. Three weeks should elapse between giving live viral vaccines and BCG or immunoglobulin. In theory the latter may suppress the development of antibodies to the vaccine but in practice this is probably not a significant issue. An interval of less than three weeks is acceptable if the alternative is to leave a subject unprotected. Live viral vaccines are also contraindicated during pregnancy and for those who are immunosuppressed or receiving systemic corticosteroids. HIV carriers, unless they are exhibiting evidence of immunosuppression, can be given live vaccines.

Adverse Reactions

The majority of reactions are confined to the site of the injection. Occasionally a delayed serum reaction occurs about ten days after the inoculation and antihistamine treatment may be indicated. Very rarely an immediate anaphylactic-type reaction can occur and ampoules of adrenaline 1:1000 should always be readily available for giving subcutaneously in the event of such a reaction. This is especially important when immunoglobulin is given.

SCABIES

This skin condition is caused by a parasitic mite, *Sarcoptes scabiei*, which burrows its way beneath the skin surface often leaving characteristic tracks. It tends to affect certain areas of the body, particularly the flexor surfaces of the wrists, web areas between the fingers, the waist, axillae and genitalia. Irritant rashes in these areas should alway raise the possibility of scabies even in the absence of the characteristic lesions. The condition usually occurs in conditions of poor social and personal hygiene and is transmitted during close bodily contact. Health care workers may contract scabies when handling patients unsuspected of having the disease.

Treatment consists of applying after a hot bath benzyl benzoate 25% emulsion or lindane 1% cream to the whole body except the head and neck. The applications should be washed off 24 hours later. The treatment should be repeated in a week's time.

CHAPTER 8

Sickness absence

The cost of providing health care services will continue to rise because of the high cost of new technology and the high staff-patient ratio required for the provision of full health care services. There are on average three staff required for each bed in a large district hospital. There is constant pressure for economies in staff to be made and many wards and departments have difficulty in providing full services when staff quotas are reduced.

Loss of staff because of sickness absence is a major concern for managers. The inevitability of this absence can be accepted when it is due to serious illness or injury. Many managers however, become frustrated and angry when they consider that absence is due to trivial or non–existent illness. The pressures upon them to continue to provide the same services with even fewer staff lead them to seek an answer to what they believe to be unjustified absence. Occupational health services are frequently required to provide explanations and solutions. Little progress will be made as long as managers regard sickness absence as entirely a medical issue and one for which they have little or no responsibility.

Whenever the problems of sickness absence are raised by management, clear and frank discussions must take place with occupational health departments. The many factors which influence this problem in both individuals and groups of employees must be identified and understood. In many instances sickness absence is due to the more trivial illnesses and to the less well defined conditions where a precise diagnosis is difficult. Because of the borderline nature of much of this minor illness there is considerable variation amongst employees regarding their criteria for remaining at work or reporting sick. The subjective judgement necessary to reach these decisions depends often on individual attitudes and on family and social traditions rather than on any absolute quality of the illness. Superimposed upon these influences there are undoubtedly factors in the working environment which contribute to sickness absence patterns. The more significant of those influences are usually the most difficult to identify or define and are those which are concerned with morale, motivation and job frustration. Factors which influence these subjective attitudes will be discussed in some detail together with the means of recording sickness absence both on an individual and a group basis.

INDIVIDUAL CHARACTERISTICS

Short spells of absence are likely to be fewer with increasing age when there is the tendency for spells of absence to be longer due to more serious or chronic illness. Women with families may be absent more often because of the need for them to remain at home with sick children and elderly dependent relatives. Cultural and social traditions also influence attitudes to minor illness. Some encourage extreme stoicism in coping with discomfort and pain while others make staying away from work the norm for the most trivial of ailments. In addition to the commitment of caring for children, which makes more demands on married women and single parents, chronic illness in one partner in a marriage may create heavy demands on the other.

Difficulties in getting to work because of distance or lack of suitable transport may also add to the likelihood of minor illness resulting in sickness absence.

Unhappiness at work and doubts about a chosen career can result in more absenteeism. In such circumstances, before finally leaving a job, a young person may suffer considerable anxiety and doubt or even depression. Table 8.1 shows the higher absenteeism amongst student nurses who gave up their training during their first year compared with the remainder of the same intake who continued their training. None of those who left did so for health reasons.

Manual workers generally have higher sickness absence rates compared with professional and managerial staff. This does not necessarily indicate that their attitude to illness or disease is different. Manual workers have few, if any, opportunities to

Table 8.1

ABSENTEEISM IN AN INTAKE OF STUDENT NURSES

	No. nurses	Total days absent	Total working days possible	% working days lost
Nurses leaving	19	571	3080	18.5
Nurses remaining	28	375	6720	5.6

modify their work when unwell. Many managerial and professional staff can make suitable adjustments to their rate of work and hours of attendance and thus offset some of the adverse effects of their illness. This is an option not available to most manual workers.

THE EFFECT OF STAFF-MANAGEMENT RELATIONSHIPS — STRUCTURE OF WORKING UNITS

There is a general trend for small working units to have lower absence rates. When the working area or unit is readily identified and constant, staff are more likely to develop a sense of responsibility and loyalty to their work colleagues and to those in charge of them. Often these factors influence individuals to remain at work or go absent when suffering from what may be called marginal illness. With the development of large district hospitals and their often remote managements, loyalty to the hospital as a whole is less likely than to the more easily recognized working unit within the hospital complex. Higher absence rates may be found in multispecialty wards where five or more consultants, each with his own junior medical staff, may have beds. In these wards regular working routines are difficult to establish as are good working relationships with the many doctors involved. Nursing staff often find the absence of a united and coordinated ward extremely frustrating and demanding. By comparison, in wards where there is only one medical team, however arduous the work, absence rates are usually lower.

Duty Rotas

The tensions and stresses of work can be offset by adequate recreation and relaxation in off-duty hours. Nursing has particular disadvantages in this respect because varying day rotas and night duty make it difficult, if not impossible, for nurses, especially those in training, to take part in regular activities outside the hospital. After a late evening duty there is usually insufficient time for mental relaxation and 'unwinding' before sleeping. When late duties are followed by early morning shifts the quality and length of sleep is often inadequate. If there is insufficient understanding and concern for these difficulties morale and motivation can suffer and sickness absence increase.

Recording and Assessment

Since 1982 self-certification has been applicable for the fourth to sixth day of absence and thereafter a doctor's certificate is required. No certificate is required for the first three days. Virtually all short-term absences will be covered by the employee's own certificate. The diagnoses are unlikely to form the basis for any accurate comparison of disease incidence. Fortunately it is the pattern of short-term absence which is most valuable in making worthwhile comparisons between units and groups of employees. In most places of employment, sick certificates are given to the immediate manager or head of department. The recording and monitoring of absence in individual working areas is therefore the responsibility of each manager. This does not allow for comparison of absence rates between departments and different categories and grades of staff. This overview can only be achieved by a separate and independent department. The personnel or occupational health units can fulfil this role. Many hospitals do not establish this central monitoring and important opportunities are lost for identifying high sickness absence rates in individual working areas or in different grades of staff. Occupational health practitioners should liaise with personnel departments to produce these figures. The salaries and wages departments are usually the best source of information for staff sickness absence details.

Sickness absence figures are often recorded as the average number of days absent per employee per year. This method of recording does not always enable accurate comparison to be made between past and present rates or between different categories and grades of staff when hours of work and holiday periods are different. It is suggested that absence is also calculated as a percentage of the total time worked per employee per year.

INVESTIGATING SICKNESS ABSENCE

Referrals to occupational health departments must follow a standard and accepted policy which is recognized by all managers and staff representatives. Before any employee is seen in the occupational health department it is essential that a referral letter from the appropriate manager or personnel department is sent with a copy to the person concerned.

The referral letter must clearly state the issue on which a medical opinion is required and must also record the extent of the sickness absence. In cases of recurrent minor absences managers may seek advice about the justification of the absences. It is strongly recommended that no opinion should be given about this as it is quite impossible and unjustified to give retrospective opinions. The occupational health practitioner should report on the present medical condition of the employee and advise whether the condition is consistent with the nature of the employment. The reply must always be given in writing with a copy sent to the employee. There are no proper circumstances in which this cannot be done. In the majority of cases of recurrent minor absences no underlying significant illness is found.

Particular conditions to look out for are chronic depression and alcohol dependency, both of which may present with a pattern of persistent minor absences. In cases of prolonged absence managers understandably need information on when the employee will be able to return to work and whether the normal occupation can be followed. If employees are still off work they should not be invited to attend the occupational health department except in a few particular circumstances. If the nature of the illness is such that a permanent disability results in a return to work being unlikely it may be helpful at a certain stage of the illness for this to be formally recognized. An initiative to effect retirement on the grounds of ill health may be in the employee's interest as well as that of the employer.

It goes without saying that great care must be exercised to ensure that the employee is able to attend the occupational health department without difficulty. In other cases of prolonged illness full recovery may be helped by a gradual return to work, or by a decision to find alternative work of a less demanding nature. Some managers are reluctant to have staff back unless able to cope fully with their normal hours of work and waiting for this stage to be reached can often result in an employee remaining off work for longer than necessary.

Another objection raised against employees returning to reduced hours for a period of time to enable full rehabilitation to take place is that it is not possible to pay a full wage for less than a full week's work. When the alternative is for the employee to continue to be off work doing no work and usually on full pay, the logic of this particular objection is difficult to follow. It is recommended that all employees who have been off sick for three or more weeks should be seen as a matter of routine in the occupational health department before returning to work. This must not be seen to be a disciplinary review but one which seeks to ensure that full recovery for the work in question has taken place. At times it may be necessary to recommend some modification of the work for a limited period.

ACCESS TO MEDICAL REPORTS ACT

This Act came into force in the UK in January 1989 and provides for patients to have access to medical reports written about them for insurance or employment purposes, by a medical practitioner who is, or has been, responsible for their medical care. It gives patients the right to see reports before they are sent to the person requesting them. It is the duty of the person seeking the report — the applicant — to inform the employee of his or her rights under this Act. An occupational health practitioner may occasionally write to a general practitioner for information about an employee who is on sick leave. In such circumstances the occupational health practitioner will be acting as the applicant under the Act. It will therefore be necessary to advise employees of their rights and also to inform the general practitioner that this advice has been given.

CHAPTER 9

Accidents — Incidence, causes and records, First aid

Injuries and accidents at work may more often be associated
with general manufacturing, mining and building industries
and less frequently with hospital employment. Large hospital
complexes of today however, have working hazards which are
comparable to those in many working situations in industry as
a whole — maintenance departments, stores, boiler houses,
laundries and kitchens being some examples. Hospital workers
in these areas not surprisingly have injury patterns which are
comparable to those of workers in similar circumstances in other
industries. Injuries more specific to health care workers more
often occur to those employees closely involved with patient
care. There are of course exceptions to this — portering, domestic
and laundry workers for example are at risk from sharps injuries
from needles and scalpel blades discarded into waste bins, refuse
bags or left in dirty linen.

RECORDS

There is no standard method for recording or assessing accident
rates in the majority of hospitals. An occupational health
department may find it necessary to initiate a system for gathering
this information to enable overall assessments to be made of the
incidence of accidents by category of staff and where they work
in the hospital. Information available on accident reports may
be filed away in employee records for use in the event of

subsequent litigation and little or no use made of the information for medical or preventative purposes. It is essential that every member of staff who sustains any significant injury completes an accident form on which are recorded the nature, cause and time of the injury. A copy of this form should routinely be sent to the occupational health department to enable relevant details to be extracted. A copy should be retained in the occupational health department and in the employee's administrative file. When records of accidents are analysed an excellent method for monitoring the safety of the hospital is available and for those who are able to establish this system the results will be rewarding. Without a centralized assessment of accidents it is not possible to detect all dangerous practices or events.

Under the Reporting of Injuries, Diseases and Dangerous Occurrences Regulations, 1985 (RIDDOR) certain accidents and dangerous occurrences at work must be reported to the Health and Safety Executive. This is a management responsibility. In some hospitals only one copy of an accident report is produced. It should be sent to the occupational health department in the first instance in order that appropriate action can be taken as soon as possible after the accident and also to ensure that the information is used to compile statistics regarding the causes and distribution of accidents among employees. If copies of the accident report are not automatically sent to management it is essential that the occupational health department liaises closely to enable the necessary information regarding accident reporting to be made available. Lack of clarity in defining the arrangements between occupational health departments and the management of hospitals often results in under-reporting of accidents among health care workers. The Reporting of Injuries, Diseases and Dangerous Occurrences Regulations require that all accidents which result in more than three days' absence must be reported within seven days of the accident. Any injury which results in a fracture of the arm, wrist, leg or ankle must also be reported and of course any injury resulting in death.

A record must be kept of all accidents which are reported either in the official Accident Book or as photocopies of form 2508 on which accidents must be reported to the Health and Safety Executive. In the event of particularly serious accidents, notification in the first instance should be by telephone. In circumstances where the accident form is sent only to the occupational health department there is a responsibility for that department to ensure that the necessary communication with the personnel department is established.

Not all incidents result in a significant injury or necessarily any injury at all; there are certain circumstances however, when such events must be reported because of their potentially dangerous nature. Some accidents may result in a sufficiently serious injury to require an immediate report to the responsible manager. An example of such an incident is illustrated by an accident to an incinerator operator at a large district general hospital who sustained severe facial burns when loading rubbish containing a discarded aerosol can into an incinerator, causing an explosion and blow back of flames. An immediate response to this type of accident is necessary in order that advice is given to all staff in the hospital of the danger of discarding aerosol cans into rubbish bags scheduled for incineration.

When recording accidents for all employees it is useful initially to relate the accident rate to different grades of staff. The following Table 9.1 shows the distribution of all accidents for a three year period for different categories of employment in a large district hospital employing 1500 staff.

The ten per cent of staff for whom no accidents were recorded included some paramedical workers and medical staff. The two groups with higher than average accident rates are the porters and laboratory technicians. Before drawing any firm conclusions from different accident rates for staff it is important to be certain

TABLE 9.1

ACCIDENT RATES IN A DISTRICT HOSPITAL FOR A THREE-YEAR PERIOD

	% of all staff	*Number of accidents*	*% of all accidents*
Administration	10	25	3.3
Catering	10	94	12.2
Domestic	18	130	17.1
Laboratory	7	126	16.4
Maintenance	6	66	8.6
Nursing	33	154	20.2
Porters	6	170	22.2
Others	10	0	0
	100	765	100

that there are similar criteria for reporting accidents amongst all staff and their managers. In certain departments accidents may be significantly under-reported because of the lack of enthusiasm and direction from management.

Having established accident rates for different grades of staff it is important to analyse their causes. Laboratory technicians will be found to sustain up to half their injuries from handling glassware, usually pipettes. Chemical burns and splashes in the eyes from various solutions are other common causes of their injuries.

Portering and domestic staff suffer a number of injuries from needles incorrectly discarded into waste bins and plastic bags. A reduction in this type of injury can be achieved by advising the appropriate wards and departments of the need to ensure that needles and scalpel blades are discarded into the appropriate sharps boxes. Not unexpectedly, one of the commoner causes of injury to catering staff are burns and scalds, followed closely by lacerations of the hands from knives used in preparing food. It is helpful and important to analyse carefully the way in which accidents occur. It is usually assumed, for example, that sharps injuries to nursing staff are inevitably a result of needles being discarded into waste bins and waste sacks instead of into the sharps boxes. A careful analysis of all sharps injuries to nurses will usually show that in fact over 50% of these injuries occur not from incorrectly discarded needles but from nurses injuring themselves when giving injections to patients. The incidents often occur just after an injection has been given and the nurse's attention is distracted.

Back injuries to the nursing staff are another major cause for concern. The reasons for these injuries are many and varied and are dealt with in more detail in the chapter on musculo-skeletal injuries. In some cases of back injury the cause and effect are clear cut in that acute back pain is experienced almost instantly after lifting or handling a patient. In other instances back symptoms may not develop until the next day and the direct relationship to a heavy spell of lifting in a ward may not be so evident. It is important however, that such events are documented on accident reports, otherwise any subsequent disabililty may not be attributable to occupation.

Accidents to which all staff are liable are falls on wet or greasy floor surfaces. The cause of this accident is probably one of the most preventable. It is common practice to wet-mop floor surfaces in hospitals and warning signs that the surfaces are wet are often inadequately displayed.

ASSAULTS BY PATIENTS

In recent years it has been the experience of most hospitals that the number of attacks by patients on staff has increased. Many hospitals have produced specific policies to advise and train staff to cope with violent incidents. The majority of assaults occur to psychiatric nurses, although staff in accident and emergency departments are also increasingly experiencing violent episodes. In one district hospital with 850 beds, out of an annual total of 108 assaults on nursing staff 71 (66%) were by psychiatric patients who comprised 10% of all in-patients. Some of these attacks may be totally unpredictable, but it has been shown that there is a tendency for assaults in psychiatric units to increase when staff changes are frequent and patients become more unsettled. This point may need to be emphasized when violent incidents are increasing. Understaffing of psychiatric wards may also expose individual staff to increased risk and danger where the understaffing may leave a nurse completely on her own in the presence of potentially violent psychotic patients.

TREATMENT OF INJURIES TO STAFF

The majority of injuries are minor and require little initial treatment. The risk of infection however from breaches of the skin, especially from needles, requires appropriate follow-up procedures and careful documentation (see Chapter 7). It is important that occupational health departments are adequately equipped to deal with these events to avoid unnecessary and inappropriate attendances at accident and emergency departments. Some occupational health practitioners do not consider that treatment should be undertaken and arrange for all staff who have had accidents, however minor, to be dealt with routinely in the accident and emergency department. In addition to avoiding unnecessary use of expensive and often overstretched accident and emergency resources there is considerable value in staff being seen and treated in occupational health departments. A golden opportunity is presented to discuss the circumstances of the accident with the injured person, to suggest safer working methods and, when necessary, to highlight the need to use protective clothing or equipment.

Depending on the occupation of the injured employee it may be necessary to liaise with the manager or supervisor to arrange temporary modification of the work while the injury resolves. It is essential to keep accurate and detailed occupational health records of every attendance. Records may be required later for medico-legal purposes, often when the employee is seeking compensation for a residual disability. Poor records can result in legitimate claims for compensation failing because of insufficient supporting medical evidence in the notes.

FIRST AID FACILITIES AND TRAINING

It is often assumed that it is unnecessary to provide and organize first aid facilities in hospital or community clinics because there are already doctors and nurses available to give treatment. The presence of accident and emergency departments may also reinforce the view that first aid will only duplicate existing cover for staff. It must be emphasized that first aid facilities are important at all places of work, including hospitals. The consequences of injuries from accidents at work may be less serious if immediate and effective first aid is given. Splashes from chemicals, acids and alkalis especially, are examples of such incidents. There are several sites on hospital premises where there are risks from these injuries. The long distances between departments in large district hospitals – half a mile from a maintenance department to an accident and emergency unit in one hospital for example — also requires that appropriate attention is paid to injuries at the place where they occur. This particularly applies to cuts, which require immediate covering, not only to reduce bleeding but also to minimize the risk of infection. Where there is any reasonable doubt about the nature and extent of an injury at work further medical attention should be sought.

It is necessary however, to keep a sense of proportion about minor skin lesions which, if they occurred to workers outside hospital premises, would be dealt with by simple first aid methods without requiring further medical attention. Adequately trained first aiders should not be required therefore to refer every single minor case of a skin breach for further medical assessment simply because the incident occurred on hospital premises. This point does not apply of course where there has been a risk of infection from patients.

The occcupational health department must ensure that all main working areas are provided with first aid boxes. The number of boxes required will depend not only on the number of staff but also on how widely dispersed some employees are when working. It may be necessary to provide a first aid box for fewer than ten workers if they are employed in a remote area of the hospital, away from other facilities. Eye wash bottles must be provided whenever chemicals are used. It is recommended that disposable bottles are provided as this will always guarantee the sterility of their contents. Bottles which are refilled are liable to be poorly maintained and run the risk of residual infection. The contents of first aid boxes must be kept as simple as possible; standard first aid dressings, a suitable variety of plasters and a few triangular bandages should be stocked. Ointments and eye drops should not be included. Supplies for stocking and refilling the boxes should be ordered from the hospital pharmacy and kept in the occupational health department, from where individual departments can obtain their supplies. This policy will ensure that there is adequate knowledge of the use of the dressings and therefore of the injuries and their causes. Each first aid box should be under the control of a named first aider.

When a first aid system is first established it is likely that there will be an insufficient number of trained first aiders available in all departments. Some occupational health practitioners may be willing and capable of giving first aid training. Many, on the other hand, are not and it is recommended that unless proper training can be guaranteed, outside experts should be invited to give training courses. The St. John's Ambulance and Red Cross organizations are usually able to provide this training and under their auspices employees can obtain a recognized first aid certificate. There is usually a charge for each employee attending the course. Where there are particular occupational health risks, splashes from chemicals in laboratories for example, it may be necessary for first aiders in those areas to have additional tuition and practice in dealing with those particular risks.

A further point should be made about giving protection against tetanus to employees sustaining minor injuries which do not require further medical attention. It should already be the policy for all employees to have protection against tetanus. Provided a sensible working arrangement is established between the occupational health unit and departments with first aid boxes, an adequate check can be kept on employees who may not already have received full protection against tetanus. First aiders should keep a careful record in the first aid book of all injuries they deal with.

CHAPTER 10

Occupational skin problems

Occupational health practitioners will from time to time see skin conditions in health care workers for which the opinion and advice of a dermatologist will be necessary. The majority of skin problems however, which are of significance occupationally, are in fact conditions which are relatively easily diagnosed and treated — eczema and dermatitis being the commonest. These conditions are important because they create difficulties in employment due to the adverse effect of many environmental factors on them, and because the skin in poor condition is more liable to be receptive to, or transmit, infection. Occupational aspects of eczema and dermatitis will be discussed, together with some other skin conditions which are fairly specifically linked to health care work.

PRE-EMPLOYMENT SELECTION

A history of eczema or dermatitis in applicants for nursing, laboratory work, catering, maintenance and domestic work must always be thoroughly reviewed and, almost without exception, the applicant must be seen. Understandably, some chronic sufferers minimize their condition when completing their health questionnaires and only when they are seen may the true extent of the problem be revealed. An occasional minor episode of eczema, limited to a small area of the face or neck, may be no contraindication to employment. Recurring outbreaks on the forearms and hands may, however, almost certainly be grounds for rejection, especially when, even in remission, the skin is dry and fissured. Students with chronic eczema of the arms and hands, who have been accepted into medical schools, may be able to undertake some branches of medicine which have little or no clinical content provided they can cope with their obligatory pre-registration posts. They will almost certainly be unfit for many clinical specialties, including surgery, obstetrics and gynaecology. Psoriasis, when limited to small areas on the elbows, may be no bar to employment, but when there are extensive lesions on the forearms, hands, face and legs, applicants are unlikely to be fit for most posts involving direct patient care.

POST-EMPLOYMENT

There are many occupational factors which may cause eczema or dermatitis. An acute condition may be caused by a one-off exposure to a particularly abrasive chemical substance. Avoidance of further exposure and treatment with local steroid or bland preparations such as aqueous cream is usually sufficient to allow resolution and early return to work. Problems may arise when the skin becomes sensitive to chemicals to which there is repeated exposure — detergent and chlorhexidine present in many liquid soap preparations, for example. The part played by trauma from repeated scrubbing up or hand washing should not be forgotten. Many people who can tolerate occasional exposure to liquid soap for hand washing, experience a breakdown of their skin when washing is necessary several times in an hour. Once detergent sensitization has developed, it may be necessary to avoid further exposure. In some situations, it may be acceptable to substitute simple soap preparations for the detergent. Sensitis-ation to chlorhexidine in nursing staff may present particular difficulties when control of infection is important. It will be necessary to discuss this aspect of the problem with the control of infection nurse or officer. Where trauma is playing an important part, as in repeated scrubbing up, even the substitution of simple soap may fail to allow the problem to resolve and only a period away from work, in addition to treatment, will allow the condition to heal. As an example, a nurse working in a special care baby unit continued to develop excoriation and erythema on her hands after changing from detergent to simple soap. The condition healed rapidly whenever she had some time away from work — albeit she continued to use ordinary soap for the less frequent social hand washing. It is extremely important to consider the part played by trauma in addition to any specific sensitiser effect of hand cleansers.

The St John's dermatology unit in London has produced a sensitivity testing kit for nurses with reactive skin problems. This can prove invaluable in identifying a specific sensitising substance, the avoidance of which may allow a nurse to continue her career.

Protective gloves

Nurses, doctors, laboratory and domestic workers are increasingly required to wear protective gloves to avoid exposure to infection. Domestic workers often wear PVC gloves throughout their working day and may develop a form of dermatitis due to excessive perspiration inside the gloves. In these cases, wearing cotton lining gloves inside the PVC ones, and changing the liners as often as necessary to avoid them becoming moist will usually control the problem.

Surgical gloves may cause dermatitis because of the irritant effect of the lubricating powder inside them. Powder-free gloves are obtainable and the provision of these may enable a nurse to continue working in theatre, when previously the substitution of PVC for latex, or vice versa, may have failed to improve matters. Where sensitisation of the rubber in standard surgical gloves has occurred, substitution of gloves made from hypo-allergenic rubber may allow resolution of the problem. Maintenance workers may suffer a breakdown of their skin because of the abrasive nature of the material of some protective gloves. Chrome leather gloves may cause dermatitis because of the coarseness of their texture and abrasiveness of the seams, and not necessarily because of any sensitising effect of the material.

Infection

In addition to the potential risk of infection from or to sufferers from eczema and dermatitis, it is important to look for other less obvious sources of infection from the skin. The minutest skin lesion infected with staphylococcal organisms on the fingers of a cook may easily be overlooked. Occasionally haemolytic streptococcal organisms may cause small erythematous lesions and be an unsuspected source of haemolytic infections on a surgical ward.

Chronic Paronychia

A low-grade but persistent form of paronychia occurs in nurses, often theatre staff, and it is most difficult to eradicate. Trauma, often from repeated scrubbing up, seems the commonest aggravating cause, so that the skin surface around the nail-base becomes cracked or fissured. A poor peripheral circulation may be an additional predisposing factor. In addition to staphylococcal organisms candida may also be found. Unless the sufferer is removed from the predisposing situation, little improvement occurs. Because infection may remain beneath the base of the nail, a recurrence is often preventable only by removal of the nail and a prolonged application of an appropriate local antibiotic.

Herpetic Whitlow

This is an infectious lesion of the skin, caused by the herpes simplex virus. Most lesions occur among nursing staff who have been handling upper respiratory tract secretions containing the virus. Postoperative care of neurosurgical patients is a common source of infection. A typical lesion begins as a painful deep-seated vesicle, usually on the thumb, index or middle finger. Other vesicles soon appear and coalesce with the lesion as a whole becoming more superficial and raised with some tissue destruction. If incised, no pus is found but only a small quantity of clear fluid. Small deep vesicles beyond the edge of the lesion characterise the condition. Bacterial infection is only secondary to the basic viral origin. If correctly diagnosed, the lesion should not be incised, but allowed to take its natural course.

At first there is pain and throbbing and a spread of the lesion for about ten days. Pain will gradually subside and the vesicles become dry and crusted. After a further seven days the crusts have usually separated with complete resolution. The condition has a similarity to the lesions of Orf on the fingers of sheep handlers. Good clinical practice and the wearing of protective gloves should minimize the risk of this infection.

Reaction to Chlorine

Physiotherapists working in hydrotherapy pools may develop patchy, irritant areas of erythema on their limbs and trunk as a result of prolonged contact with chlorine during their treatment sessions. The reactions may occur not only because of the length of exposure to chlorine but also as a result of the chlorine content of the water being too high, several instances of which are known to the authors. The chlorine levels in hydrotherapy pools should be checked daily and kept between 1 and 1.5 parts per million. Where cases of skin reactions have occurred in physiotherapists in hydrotherapy pools, chlorine levels of between 3 and 3.5 parts per million have been reached. Removal from hydrotherapy pool work and maintenance of correct chlorine levels will usually control the problem, but in rare cases it may be necessary to avoid hydrotherapy work altogether, to prevent recurring problems.

Boils and Minor Staphylococcal Skin Lesions

Where such lesions are present on exposed parts of the skin, it will be necessary for most employees to be off work until resolution has occurred. Where the lesions are on areas of the body which are completely covered — the trunk, for example — it may be acceptable for most staff to remain at work. Ultimate decisions on these issues will be the responsibility of the control of infection officer, whose views and advice must always be sought.

CHAPTER 11

Back pain

The statistics about back pain are too well known to repeat here and the justification for including a separate chapter is that it is such a common problem, particularly amongst nursing staff, that special consideration seems appropriate; the same applies to skin disease which has also been given a chapter of its own.

Although back pain is not peculiar to nursing staff, they are the group amongst whom it seems most common and because they are numerically the largest section of health care workers, more nurses with bad backs are seen than anyone else. The antecedents are simple; nurses are required to undertake manual handling tasks of a magnitude which no other section of the working population would tolerate for a moment. A visit to any ward will cause the visitor to reflect not that it is surprising that so many nurses develop bad backs but how amazing that some do *not*.

Lifting patients up and down beds, in and out of beds, into and out of chairs, to and from the ward toilets, in and out of baths and onto and off toilets is achieved with no consideration as to the congruity between the nurse and the patient, or between the pairs of nurses lifting together; the ergonomics of the work is appalling and lifting aids are seldom if ever available. Although it is usual for some training in lifting techniques to be given to student nurses, it is difficult to put theory into practice when the conditions under which the nurse has to lift are not conducive to it.

Back pain has important consequences both to the nurse and to the employer. For the nurse it may mean days or weeks of discomfort; it will result in time lost from work and if this is more than a few days a year, the postponement of qualification; in a number of cases, it may be necessary for the nurse to leave the profession and seek other work. For the employer the result of back pain means disruption on the wards and clinics and a considerable financial penalty because of the need to employ agency staff to cover for staff who are absent and because of potentially large awards which may have to be paid by way of compensation to those who are forced to leave the profession. But despite this, there is a considerable inertia to take any positive steps to investigate ways of preventing the occurrence of back pain or rehabilitating those who suffer from it quickly back to work.

PREVENTION

Most back pain is muscular in origin and there is some evidence that exercises designed to strengthen the muscles of the back, especially the erector spinae are successful in reducing the prevalence of back pain to some degree. Nurses need to be trained to carry out the exercises by someone with the appropriate skills and this is most often a physiotherapist or a physical training instructor; the training needs to be reinforced at frequent intervals — it is hopeless to give one course of training at an early stage in a nurses' career and assume that this will suffice — and the exercises must be done regularly and not only during or just after an episode of pain. To employ someone with the special responsibility of training nurses (and others) to exercise and to lift properly has been shown to be cost-effective and if occupational health departments could cajole their authorities into making such appointments, there is no doubt that the investment would be more than returned in the saving of time lost and of agency fees.

Pre-employment assessment has little to offer in the way of preventing back pain. As we mention elsewhere, it was once the policy not to accept young women for training if they were either unusually short or unusually tall; the rationale for these restrictions seems somewhat obscure and may never have been more than a subjective whim. Generally one would not place height restrictions on entrants into nurse training unless the deviation from normal was particularly gross. Some departments like to assess back mobility before accepting applicants as fit for training but the utility of this procedure has not been demonstrated; special investigations such as measuring the diameter of the spinal canal with ultrasound were much mooted at one time but more recent evidence does not suggest that they have much to offer.

Probably the only grounds for rejecting a candidate would be if there was a long history of back pain or a serious injury to the back or of an established spondylarthropathy such as ankylosing spondylitis.

So far as ergonomics are concerned, it is unlikely ever that lifting aids will be generally available but beds on which the height can be adjusted are, and should be used as standard. There should be enough room around the beds and in toilets and bathrooms so that the nurses can attend to their patients in comfort and without having to contort themselves into postures which put them at even greater risk of a back injury. The floors of all clinical departments should be of a non-slip material to avoid accidental falls. When wheelchairs or trolleys are used, it is important to ensure that the brakes are securely on. Finally, it is surely time that nurses were dressed more appropriately for their work and followed the example of their colleagues in North America who wear trousers as standard.

INVESTIGATION OF BACK PAIN

Although the majority of back pain seen by the occupational physician will be muscular in origin it is important to make a careful examination in each case in order to exclude other causes which may need referral to another consultant. None would be likely to occur commonly but disc lesions with root involvement, spondylarthropathies such as ankylosing spondylitis and other conditions such as spondylolisthesis must occasionally be encountered. Amongst the older segment of the population osteoarthritis affecting the facet joints is common and may give rise to back pain as may metastatic disease.

Unless there are positive clinical grounds for doing so, such as a history of constant, increasing pain, an X-ray of the lumbar spine should not be requested since it will invariably be normal or show some abnormality such as spondylolysis which is merely a confounder. It is often difficult to maintain this counsel of perfection since many back pain sufferers have a touching belief that the X-ray will reveal the 'cause' of their pain and may become extremely insistent; since none of us is perfect, the tempation to accede to such a request may be too great to resist and in rare instances, the procedure does indeed have some therapeutic advantage especially where some abnormality is actually shown to be present.

TREATMENT AND REHABILITATION

The treatment of back pain is not a simple matter and those who have the condition are often heartily discouraged by the length of time which resolution of their pain may take. Much of the advice which is given to those with back pain is frankly misleading and tends usually to prolong rather than shorten the period of recovery. For example, bed rest and inactivity are frequently counter-productive in the absence of neurological signs as might happen with an acute prolapsed disc, for example, and a regime of proper exercises is much to be preferred. All cases of back pain should be assessed by the occupational physician and we recommend that they devise rehabilitation programmes which will certainly ensure that time lost from work will be minimized. In most hospitals rehabilitation is undertaken with the help of the physiotherapy department although there may be a conflict between service requirements and treatment of staff. As we have mentioned already, it is cost-effective for the occupational health department to have their own specialist in lifting and handling and it is clearly advantageous that this person should be a physiotherapist who could run rehabilitation sessions for staff with back pain. If this is not feasible, then some consideration should be given to devoting some clinical sessions to the services of a physician with a special interest in orthopaedics or sports medicine; from personal experience we are able to testify to the great value of having such a person as part of the occupational health team.

CHAPTER 12

Pregnancy and health care employment

The majority of staff in hospitals — between 75 and 80% — are women, of whom approximately 75% are of childbearing age. In addition to some of the physical and chemical hazards which may adversely affect fetal development, such as cytotoxic drugs, radiation, anaesthetic gases and viruses, other factors relating to stress and organization of the working environment will be discussed. Many of the causes of abnormal development of embryos inevitably exert their effect at an early stage in the developmental process. It follows therefore that women who may become pregnant must be protected at all times from factors in the environment which are potentially damaging to the fetus, and not only when pregnancy is diagnosed. By the time pregnancy is diagnosed, it may be too late to avoid damage to the fetus. Before reviewing specific factors adversely affecting pregnancy, some general issues will be discussed.

It is generally considered that during a normal healthy pregnancy women should not be precluded from working up to eleven weeks from the date of delivery. It is important however, to avoid unduly heavy work and work which requires prolonged standing. Undue tiredness may be a very marked feature during some or all of pregnancy, particularly for women who are running homes and who already have children. It is generally recommended therefore, that shift work and irregular hours should be avoided. It may be difficult for many nurses who become pregnant to avoid such irregular hours. This is particularly true of nurses in training. Student nurses who become pregnant may not always have planned to have a child, but in spite of this may wish to continue with the pregnancy and to complete their training at the same time. Occupational health practitioners can give considerable help and encouragement to a student nurse who intends both to continue her pregnancy and training, by seeing her at regular intervals for counselling and general support. In many cases, in spite of trying to succeed with the dual commitment, a student nurse finds it impossible to cope and has to give up her training.

It is important that qualified nursing staff are also seen periodically in the occupational health department, to ensure that they are not experiencing undue difficulties or tiredness in remaining at work. It may be possible to help them modify some aspect of their work which may be causing particular difficulties, if there is adequate liaison with management. Unfortunately, many families have heavy financial commitments which require both partners to remain at work and much anxiety is generated at the prospect of one of them having to stop earning. Most pregnant staff are not anxious, for this reason, to stop work before the 29th week of pregnancy. General practitioners and antenatal clinics will be giving more specific advice, including the need to avoid alcohol and smoking during pregnancy. It may be helpful, however, to reinforce these points, Not all hospitals have smoking policies and attention should be paid to staff who are exposed to passive smoking in their offices.

General Physical Trauma

It is almost impossible to undertake normal nursing duties without having to lift or support patients. Full nursing duties therefore are not in general compatible with continuing to work during pregnancy. It may be possible however, if some of the heavier aspects of nursing can be excluded, for employment to continue up to the 29th week of pregnancy.

Radiation

There is no evidence that non-ionizing radiation from ultrasound instruments and microwaves is injurious to the fetus. There is also no established evidence that working with VDUs exposes a mother or fetus to any hazard. However, considerable anxiety and concern has been generated regarding the use of VDUs during pregnancy. It spite of reassurance, some pregnant women remain apprehensive about working with a VDU. It may be justified in some circumstances, therefore, to recommend alternative work, to avoid undue anxiety.

The potential risk of exposure to ionizing radiation exists mainly for those who work in X-ray departments or radiotherapy units. In properly protected radiotherapy and X-ray units there should be no risk to a pregnancy and regular monitoring of radiation levels should ensure that this is always so. Anxiety, however, may exist and it is recommended that each case should be assessed carefully before making any automatic rules about remaining at work in these areas during pregnancy, even though levels of radiation are being monitored and are known to be safe. Other factors should also be considered. The wearing of heavy lead aprons can be tiring for anyone, but particularly so during pregnancy. It may therefore be difficult for pregnant staff working in X-ray departments to comply with all the safety regulations. Mobile X-ray machines are liable to cause scattering of radiation and it is recommended that pregnant staff should avoid using this particular type of apparatus. In dental departments it is not always possible to control the exposure of assistants to radiation, particularly where it is necessary for some patients to be supported when being X-rayed. It is important for dental assistants to be aware that, should they intend to become pregnant, they should avoid working in these departments unless protected by lead aprons.

Anaesthetic Gases

A number of studies have suggested an association between congenital abnormalities and spontaneous abortion, in women who have been exposed to anaesthetic gases before or during their pregnancy, with the increased risk of spontaneous abortion especially in the first three months of pregnancy. Other studies have thrown doubts as to whether the increase in spontaneous abortion relates to exposure to anaesthetic gases, suggesting that the higher rates relate more to tensions and stresses of some occupations in theatres and to the amount of alcohol consumption. Staff who work in theatres, who are considering becoming pregnant, should be aware that it may be advisable for them to seek alternative posts.

Cytotoxic Drugs

Animal studies have indicated that exposure to these drugs can result in mutagenic and teratogenic changes. All hospitals should have policies for the safe handling of cytotoxic drugs, which will ensure that these drugs are made up in pharmacies where there is proper exhaust ventilation, and not on wards or in outpatients. The drugs should only be administered by staff who have been adequately instructed and trained in their use. In some hospitals, cytotoxic drugs may still be handled and made up by staff in wards or outpatient departments, and administered without special training or instruction. It has been shown, although the numbers studied were small, that there is an increase in fetal abnormalities amongst female health care workers who have at some time in the past handled cytotoxic drugs. It should perhaps be pointed out that males who have been exposed to cytotoxic drugs may also have had the potential to suffer the mutagenic effects of the drugs and therefore influence adversely an ensuing pregnancy.

Infectious Diseases

It is well known that exposure of susceptible subjects to the rubella virus in early pregnancy may result in fetal abnormalities. No health care worker should experience such a tragedy, because all should be screened for rubella susceptibility when they first start work in hospitals or community clinics. An occupational health department must always ensure that women of childbearing age, working with patients, are not at risk from this particular hazard.

Other viruses may also affect the fetal development. There is an increased likelihood of staff being exposed to viruses when working on children's wards. Staff in these circumstances who are contemplating pregnancy should have the opportunity to avoid working in paediatric units prior to conception and during the early months of pregnancy.

From time to time questions are raised about the effect on pregnancy of exposure to the cytomegalovirus. For all practical purposes, this virus does not have any occupational significance or risk for health care workers during pregnancy.

Human Immunodeficiency Virus (HIV)

The risk of the human immunodeficiency virus being transmitted from an infected patient to a health care worker following a sharps injury, has been assessed at approximately a 1 in 250 chance. Individual responses and attitudes to this degree of risk vary considerably — depending, amongst other things, on the seriousness of the consequences of the risk and whether it is the person at risk or their adviser who is making the assessment. Obvious as these observations may be, they are highly relevant when a health care worker who is pregnant sustains a sharps injury from an HIV positive patient. The anxiety felt by an individual in these circumstances is compounded by the knowledge that, if infected, the virus will almost certainly be passed on to the unborn child. The extreme seriousness of the consequences of the risk is likely to make the odds of 1 in 250 cause for maximum concern and anxiety for the injured person. Testing for HIV antibodies will not afford an immediate solution, because antibodies will not appear as a rule until three months after the incident and possibly not for as long as a year later. The question of terminating the pregnancy will become an immediate issue. There can be few areas of medical practice which require more skilled and experienced assessment in order that the right guidance and advice is given. A final decision should be made only after the most experienced counselling has been provided. Whether it is decided to continue with the pregnancy or not, the person concerned will require a great deal of care and counselling in the ensuing months.

It is important that staff who are intending to become, or who already are, pregnant should not work where there is an increased risk of there being HIV positive patients — sexually transmitted disease, drug dependency or infectious disease units, for example.

Organic Solvents

There may be some association with exposure to solvents and an increased tendency to develop pre-eclampsia. There has been speculation that this may be related to the association of renal disease and solvent exposure. Doubts remain, however, about the certainty of this relationship. It serves nevertheless as a reminder of the need at all times for strict control of the use of solvents and for the proper use of extractor cabinets whenever solvents are handled.

CHAPTER 13

The sick doctor

There may be some surprise that of all the health professionals only doctors have been chosen for discussion in a separate chapter. There are, however, some good reasons for this as we hope to make clear. Doctors tend to be less well managed than other staff in the health service, their work is less well monitored and there are seldom any procedures for overseeing their sick leave or for arranging that they be seen to assess their fitness to work after prolonged or frequent absence from work. Doctors also tend to be the group who invariably slip through the occupational health net; it is seldom that they are seen before they are appointed or when they take up a new appointment.

Doctors frequently have a cynical view of the competence of other practitioners and it is common for them to treat themselves (including the prescription of medicines) and their families. They rarely consider occupational health practitioners as having much to offer them and in our experience rarely consult their occupational physician colleagues if they do have a problem which might affect their work. Some rationalize their attitude by sheltering behind the cloak of confidentiality; after all it may be difficult to discuss a drinking problem with a colleague who might next be met in a committee or over the lunch table. Doctors seldom consider that similar problems may be encountered by other members of staff or by management who generally do not find such considerations a bar to taking what their occupational health department has to offer.

It may be difficult for other health care workers to sympathize or empathize with these attitudes but they are real and there is little prospect of them being overcome in the near future. There is one other important reason for treating the health of doctors separate from others and that is that (with few exceptions) it is the doctor who has the ultimate responsibility for the investigation and treatment of patients; doctors subject patients to uncomfortable and potentially dangerous invasive procedures; and they recommend and sometimes persuade patients to undergo operations and to take drugs which may have serious side-effects. It is therefore essential that their judgement is not impaired or their competence adversely affected by physical or mental illness or by the abuse of drugs or alcohol.

MANAGEMENT AND THE DOCTOR

The relationship between management and the doctor is imprecise and is almost wilfully kept that way by the doctors themselves who would like to think of themselves as free agents in the health service. Consultants are managerially accountable to the District General Manager and profesionally to the Regional Medical Officer. However, with many working part-time and for a number of different authorities, and with some being employed by academic institutions although carrying out most of their work in the health service, it is difficult in practice to manage them effectively on a day-to-day basis. Junior doctors tend to consider themselves as working for a 'firm' but the consultant (or consultants) who head their firm is in no sense their manager.

Many of the problems in dealing adequately with the sick doctor stem from this fundamental weakness in the management structure and from the reluctance of those who do have the responsibility to take steps to intervene when something clearly is wrong. It is embarrassing to confront colleagues, especially those who may be very senior or very eminent to suggest that their standard of work is falling off or that their health may be acting to the detriment of their practice. Occupational health physicians suffer from this no less than other doctors and many do not relish in the slightest having to deal with other doctors; and there is precious little in their own training which helps them to cope with their own feelings of inadequacy in this respect.

IDENTIFYING THE SICK DOCTOR

There has been a substantial body of research into sick doctors (or impaired physicians as they are known in North America) and it is clear that doctors enjoy better physical health but poorer mental health than those in other professions. Their rate of suicide is especially high and this has been confirmed by many studies. For example, it is twice as high as in the general population and appears to be higher in those who practise in a country which is not the place of their birth. Dependence on alcohol or on other drugs is also more prevalent than amongst other occupational groups and is particularly high in anaesthetists and general practitioners. This is reflected in the referrals to those programmes which have been set up to help sick doctors. In both the UK and North America only a handful of those who have been dealt with have a physical rather than a psychiatric illness.

By contrast with the wealth of information about their psychiatric state very little is known about the prevalence of physical illness or disability amongst doctors or about the amount of time lost from work. This is clearly an area where more research should be undertaken.

PRESENT MECHANISMS

When a doctor becomes sick in this country there is no accepted mechanism by which he or she can be referred to an occupational physician as any other sick employee would be; indeed, as has already been noted, there is a reluctance to go down this route both on the part of management and the doctor concerned. Collusion between the sick doctor and his colleagues is all too frequent and in most hospitals of any size there is at least one doctor who is known by his colleagues to drink too much or to be psychiatrically ill but who choose to do nothing but gossip about it, or if they work closely with him complain of the extra work load which has come their way. Open and frank confrontation is the exception rather than the rule. When asked why this is so, some doctors will say that to do otherwise would be to offend professional etiquette and others invoke the Hippocratic convention which places a duty on physicians to regard all others in the profession as their brothers (or sisters), except it seems when it comes to caring about their health.

When a referral is made to the occupational health department the occupational physician is often not given a proper background to the case. For example he may not be told that a drink problem is suspected or that the patient's colleagues have long considered that he is unable to carry out properly his duties and responsibilities. The hope and expectation is that the occupational physician will declare the patient unfit for work thus sparing anyone else the unpleasant task of raising the issue of work performance themselves.

The best known informal system of dealing with sick doctors is through the so-called Three Wise Men. These are a group of senior doctors within the hospital, usually the Chairman of the Medical Executive Committee and two others, one of whom is a psychiatrist. The three wise men may directly approach a doctor whom they think may be in trouble, or referral may be made to them by colleagues. No audit is made of the system and so there is no means of knowing how effective it is nor how frequently occupational health professionals may be called in to help deal with the situation.

There are a number of voluntary schemes to which sick doctors themselves may have recourse and ten or so self-help groups. A national counselling scheme was set up for sick doctors in the UK in 1985 and doctors may either refer themselves or seek advice about colleagues. The scheme is entirely confidential and most of those giving help are psychiatrists. Unfortunately, the effectiveness of this service is completely unknown because it is so secret that there is no means of monitoring outcome. This seems to be taking the tenets of confidentiality to absurd lengths and to ensure that the service can neither be changed nor improved.

The General Medical Council has a Health Committee which can advise doctors who have been brought to the attention of the GMC and who are thought to be in need of medical attention (again, almost invariably psychiatric attention). The Committee has no powers to require doctors to seek medical attention but it can make remaining on the Register dependent upon doing so or it can defer ruling in a case until the result of medical assessment or treatment is known. This scheme does seem to be effective in so far that many of those who are dealt with by the committee remain in practice; the principal disadvantage of this scheme, however, is that it can deal only with doctors whose performance has deteriorated to such a degree that their capability to practice has been brought in to question.

In the US some states have a 'sick physician statute' which defines the inability of a physician to practise medicine with reasonable skill and safety to his patients because of one or more illnesses which are listed in the statute; these illnesses invariably include abuse of alcohol or drugs. If probable cause is shown that a physician is impaired then he or she is required to submit to medical examination; prior consent to this examination is deemed to have been given by the physician by using his licence to practise and by the annual renewal of the licence. In some states it is mandatory for other physicians to report to the licensing board any information which may show that another doctor is unfit to practise.

The American Medical Association has sponsored an impaired physicians' movement which attempts in the words of one author 'to rescue faltering physicians from the wasteland of physical and emotional impairment'. Each state makes its own arrangements in this regard but one of the best known is the impaired physicians' programme of the Medical Association of Georgia which had 1,000 physicians referred to it between 1975 and 1986. The Californian Medical Association also has a well-known programme which was established after a change in Californian law which permitted sick doctors to enter treatment rather than immediately face disciplinary action. It was found that sick doctors came to light and were treated much more quickly when the due process of law was not involved and that the great majority were able to continue in practice whilst undergoing treatment. The significant feature of all the American programmes is that they are closely monitored and the outcome of treatment is known.

SUGGESTED METHODS FOR TREATING THE SICK DOCTOR

There are undoubtedly many factors which contribute towards mental illness in doctors, for that is what we are principally considering here. The career structure itself has been recognized as one important stressor with insecurity of tenure, the frequent need to move and a prolonged period of postgraduate training with no certainty as to eventual outcome. Long hours, poor conditions of work and poor inter-personal relations with consultants, make the lot of the junior doctors particularly stressful although no-one has yet managed to devise a system by which their long hours can be reduced and yet still gain the unique experience of those early post-qualification years.

Doctors should not be encouraged to believe that they merit special treatment from their employers for, certainly with regard to their own health, special treatment generally means worse treatment. It is our view that doctors should be accorded the same care and consideration as all other employees within the health service. If this is to be achieved then a system for their effective management must be devised, since health and safety at work is a management responsibility, and reliance must be placed on formal and not informal methods of coping with a doctor who becomes unfit to work. In general practice there would need to be an agreement that the partners were responsible for each other and that where there was a cause for concern, referral to a local occupational physician would be an acceptable course of action. Family Practitioner Committees could circulate their practitioners with names of occupational physicians who would agree to act in this capacity.

Who should manage doctors is not a matter on which we feel competent to judge except to note that some consideration should perhaps be given to making this a responsibility of clinical directors when they are appointed.

What we are clear about, however, is that doctors should expect that their occupational health needs will be met and it should be expected that they in turn will conform to those requirements which pertain to all staff. Thus, some form of pre-employment assessment should be the norm; this is particularly important in the case of doctors who may suffer from a physical impairment, who may have a past history of physical or mental illness or who may have required an unusual amount of sick leave in the past. In practice it is easy enough to ensure that pre-employment assessment is made by not issuing a contract without the advice from the occupational health department that there is no medical reason not to do so.

Once in employment, pharmacies and laboratories should make it an absolute rule that they will not dispense drugs or carry out tests which are requested by individuals for themselves or their families, or which are requested by other doctors on behalf of a colleague unless that colleague is a patient or unless it is the occupational physician who makes the request.

Some regular monitoring of the health of doctors at work may now be necessary under the terms of the COSHH regulations in the UK; for example, those physicians who regularly undertake endoscopy may be sufficiently exposed to glutaraldhyde to require regular health surveillance. It may also be thought desirable that older doctors working in high technology medicine should have an annual or biennial examination to ensure that there are no medical contra-indications to them continuing with this work.

We subscribe to the view that all doctors have a duty to ensure that their colleagues are fit to practise their art and that this duty to the public overrides any other considerations. With a proper management structure, frequent bouts of sick leave or other classic indicators of ill health or dependence on drugs or alcohol should be quickly apparent and the norm then should be a referral to the occupational physician with a proper letter which sets out the reasons for the referral and what is expected of it. It may be felt that referral to an occupational physician in the same hospital is too sensitive, in which case it would be relatively easy to set up a reciprocal system whereby occupational physicians would see sick doctors in each other's districts.

It is notable that in discussions about treating the sick doctor, occupational health physicians are generally not considered by their colleagues, and especially their psychiatric colleagues, to have any role to play at all. This is completely to misunderstand the function of the occupational physician which is not to enter into the treatment of the individual but to do what they are good at; assess the ability and capacity of others to continue in their work and to make proper and appropriate referral to outside agencies with the collaboration of the individual's general practitioner where they have one.

Two final points here. If occupational physicians are to retain (some may even say gain) credibility in the eyes of their colleagues, then they must be seen to be able to deal competently and well with sick doctors and many would not be reluctant to admit that this is an area of their work which they do not do best; clearly this should form part of the training of an occupational physician. Finally, we feel that a great deal more research needs to be undertaken into the prevalence of illness in the medical profession and the effect this has on work practices.

MEDICAL STUDENTS

One way to ensure both that doctors look more favourably on the occupational health service and that they use it when they need it, is through the education of medical students. Medical students receive little enough formal training in occupational medicine during their course, two or three hours at best if they are lucky, and given the insatiable demands on their time, this is not going to be improved upon. However, since the COSHH regulations now require all those who are exposed to substances hazardous to health to be given sufficient training to understand the nature of the risks involved and how they can be minimized, this should provide an opportunity for the occupational health department in teaching hospitals to become involved with students in the matter of their own health and safety.

As well as concentrating on the strict tenets of the COSHH regulations, the training session could also touch upon the other occupational hazards which will present themselves during the normal working life of a doctor. If the department also provides the occupational health service to the students, this will give an added opportunity for education and the build-up of confidence in the staff. The aim would be to develop in the students an attitude of mind which would lead them automatically to turn to the occupational health department for help and advice with all work related problems.

Some ill health may be prevented if more attention were given to the selection of young men and women for medical training. At present it is carried out on a very amateur basis and compares extremely badly compared with the way in which, for example, potential officers are recruited into the armed services. Neither top grades in 'A'-levels nor the ability unerringly to put a rugby ball between two uprights necessarily fits an individual for a career in medicine and selection procedures must be adapted to ensure, so far as is practicable, that those chosen are well motivated and are likely to be able to withstand the rigours both of the training and the subsequent life as a doctor. Some research has been undertaken to assess selection procedures but it is not evident that the results of these studies have led to any re-evaluation of procedures.

Sources of information and help for medical and social problems

The functions and purpose of most of the associations and societies listed are indicated by their titles. Where this is not so, a brief explanatory note is included.

Classification to help reference has been made under the following headings:

Abortion

AIDS

Alcohol problems

Anorexia — see under Psychiatric problems

Bereavement

Blindness and partially sighted

Child and parental problems, including child abuse

Counselling

Disablement

Drugs

Elderly — see also Retirement

Family planning

Gambling

General dental and medical practitioners

Health education

Hearing problems

Homosexuality

Marital problems

Medical conditions — congenital and acquired — see also under Psychiatric and Mental handicap; and Women's problems

Mental handicap

Psychiatric illness

Psychotherapy

Rape

Retirement

Single parents

Smoking

Women's problems — social and medical

Abortion
British Pregnancy Advisory Service
tel: 071–222 0985
7 Belgrave Road,
London,
SW1V 1QB

Miscarriage Association
tel: 0924 85515

Post-abortion Counselling Service
tel: 071-263 7599

Pregnancy Advisory Service
tel: 081-891 6833
The Cottage,
17 Rosslyn Road,
East Twickenham,
Middlesex,
TW1 2AR

AIDS
AIDS Healthline — ask for AIDS
  tapes
tel: 0392 59191

Body Positive
support for those who are HIV
  positive
tel: 071-833 2971

Frontliners — people with AIDS
tel: 071-831 0330

Mainliners — drug users with HIV
P.O. Box 125,
London, SW9 8EF

National AIDS Helpline
• Access to trained advisers, and
  information on local helplines
  and groups
  tel: 0800 567123 — 24
  hours
• To obtain free booklets
  tel: 0800 555777 — 24
  hours

Terrence Higgins Trust
tel: 071-242 1010 (Helpline)

N.B. Look in telephone directory or
in general practitioners waiting
room for information about local
services and AIDS counsellors.
Also contact nearest sexually
transmitted disease (STD) clinic or
Health Education Department.

Alcohol Problems
ACCEPT
tel: 071-381 3155

AL-ANON — help for families of
  those with drink problems.
tel: 071-403 0888
61 Great Dover Street,
London, SE1 4YF

ALATEEN — support for young
  people with dependency problems,
  or whose relatives are affected.
tel: 071-403 0888 (24 hours)
61 Great Dover Street,
London, SE1 4YF

Alcoholics Anonymous — main
  centre for reference
tel: 0904 644026

Alcoholics Anonymous — general
  service office
Stonebow House,
Stonebow,
York, YO1 2NJ
Other main centres:
London   071-352 3001
Scotland   041-221 9027
N. Ireland   0232 681084
Wales South West   0222 373771
Wales West   0994 5282
Also look in telephone directory for
  local office.

Alcohol Concern
tel: 071-833 3471
305 Gray's Inn Road,
London, WC1X 8QF

Alcohol Concern Wales
tel: 0222 48800
Brunel House,
2 Fitzallan Road,
Cardiff, CF2 1EB

Medical Council on Alcoholism
tel: 071-487 4445
1 St Andrews Place,
London, NW1 4LB

Northern Ireland Council on Alcohol
tel: 0232 664434
40 Elmwood Avenue,
Belfast, BT9 6AZ

Scottish Council on Alcohol
tel: 041-333 9677
137/145 Sauchiehall Street,
Glasgow, G2 2EW

Bereavement
Bereaved Parents Helpline
tel: 0279 412745
6 Canons Gate,
Harlow,
Essex, CM20 1QE

Cruse
Bereavement Care
tel: 081-940 4818
Cruse House,
126 Sheen Road,
Richmond,
Surrey, T9 1UR

The Samaritans
Central London — 071-439 2224
see local telephone directory

Blindness and partially sighted
Braille Correspondence Club
tel: 0632 32850 Ext. 6320
Room 57, Social Services
   Department,
Civic Centre, Barvas Bridge,
Newcastle, NE1 8PA

National Deaf Blind and Rubella
   Association
tel: 071-278 1005
311 Gray's Inn Road,
London, WC1X 8PT

National Federation of the Blind
tel: 0924 892146
Unity House,
Smyth Street,
Wakefield,
W. Yorks, WF1 1ER

Partially Sighted Society
tel: 0302 68998
Queen's Road,
Doncaster,
Yorks, DN1 2NX

Tape Correspondence Club — help
   for visually handicapped to
   communicate by tapes
tel: 05806 2213
19 Turners Avenue,
Tenterden,
Kent, TH30 6QL

**Children and Parental Problems,
   including Child Abuse**
Child — help for infertile couples
tel: 071-790 9686
367 Wandsworth Road,
London, SW8 2JJ

Childline — physical or sexual abuse
tel: 0800 1111 (free)

Church of England Children's
   Society
tel: 071-837 4299
Edward Rudolf House,
Margery Street,
London, WC1X 0JL

Contact a Family — self help
   organization for families with
   handicapped children
tel: 071-222 2695/2461

16 Stratton Ground,
London, SW1P 2HP

Cot Death Research
tel: 0836 219010 (24 hour
helpline)
8A Alexandra Parade,
Weston-super-Mare,
BS23 1QT

Crysis — help for parents with
babies and toddlers who cry
excessively and have disturbed
nights
tel: 071-404 5011
c/o BM Crysis
London, WC1N 3XX

Daycare Trust and the National
Childcare Campaign
tel: 071-405 5617/8
Wesley House,
4 Wild Court,
London, WC2B 5AU

Gingerbread
Help for one-parent families
tel: 071-240 0953
35 Wellington Street,
London, WC2E 7BN

Grandparents Federation
Advice on rights to see
grandchildren
tel: 0279 37145
Noreen Tingle
78 Cook's Spinney,
Harlow,
Essex, CM20 3BL

Handicapped Independent Parent
Association
Help for disabled parents with
children
tel: 04023 49675
8 Lavender Close,
Harold Hill,
Romford,

Essex, RM3 8AU

Incest Crisis Line
tel: 081-422 5100/890 4732
32 Newbury Close,
Northolt,
Middlesex, UB5 4JF

Incest Lifeline
tel: 0793 731286

In Touch — contact for parents of
children with similar problems
tel: 061-962 4441
10 Norman Road,
Sale,
Cheshire, M33 3DF

National Childbirth Trust
tel: 081-992 8637
Alexandra House,
Oldham Terrace,
London, W3 6NH

OPUS — Organization for Parents
Under Stress
tel: 081-645 0469
106 Godstone Road,
Whyteleaf,
Surrey, CR3 0EB

Parents Anonymous London
tel: 071-263 8918
6–9 Manor Gardens,
London, N7 6LA

Parents' Enquiry – for parents with
worries about homosexual
teenagers
tel: 081-698 1815
16 Honley Road,
Catford,
London, SE6 2HZ

Parents Lifeline — help for parents
with critically ill or dying children
tel: 071-263 2265 (24 hours)
Station House,
73D Stapleton Hall Road,

London, N4 3QF

Parent to Parent — information on
    adoption
tel: 0327 60295
Lower Boddington,
Daventry,
Northampton, NN11 6YB

Reach
Children with artificial limbs
tel: 0460 61578
13 Park Terrace,
Cromchard,
Chard,
Somerset, TA20 1LA

STEPS
Support for families with children
    with congenital abnormalities of
    the lower limbs
tel: 061-747 7014
8 Princess Road,
Urmston,
Manchester, M31 3SS

The Cot Death Society
tel: 0635 523756
4 Mansell Drive,
Wash Common,
Newbury,
Berks, RG14 6TE

The Foundation for the Study of
    Infant Deaths
tel: 071-235 1721
15 Belgrave Square,
London, SW1X 8PS

The National Childminding
    Association
tel: 081-464 6164
8 Masons Hill,
Bromley,
Kent, BR2 9EY

The Scottish Cot Death Trust
tel: 041-357 3946

Royal Hospital for Sick Children,
Yorkhill,
Glasgow, G3 8SJ

Counselling
British Association for Counselling
Advice and information about local
    qualified counsellors
tel: 0788 78328
37A Sheep Street,
Rugby,
Warwickshire,
CV21 2BX

CHAT — Counselling Help and
    Advice Together — for all nurses
tel: 071-629 3870 or 071-409
    3333
Royal College of Nursing,
20 Cavendish Square,
London, W1M 0AB

Young People's Counselling Service
tel: 071-435 7111 Ext. 337
Tavistock Centre,
120 Belsize Lane,
London, NW3 5BA

Disablement
Disabled Drivers Association
tel: 081-692 7141; 0508 41449
18 Creekside,
London, SE8 3DZ

Mobility International
Help to contact others with similar
    disabilities
tel: 071-403 5688
228 Borough High Street,
London, SE1 1JX

Queen Elizabeth's Foundation for the
    Disabled.
Help with education, careers,
    accommodation and holidays.
tel: 0372 842204
Leatherhead Court,

Woodlands Road, Leatherhead,
Surrey, KT22 0BN

Riding for the Disabled
tel: 0203 696510
Avenue 'R', National Agricultural
  Centre,
Kenilworth,
Warwickshire, CV8 2LY

Royal Association for Disability and
  Rehabilitation (RADAR)
tel: 071-637 5400
25 Mortimer Street,
London, W1N 8AB

Swimming Clubs for the
  Handicapped
tel: 0273 559470
219 Preston Drive,
Brighton,
Sussex, BN1 6FL

Vocal
Help with speech and language
  difficulties
tel: 071-274 4029
336 Brixton Road,
London, SW9 7AA

Welsh Sports Association for the
  Disabled
tel: 0222 566281
Rockwood Hospital,
Llandaff,
Cardiff, CF5 2YN

Drugs
Families Anonymous
Mutual support group for friends
  and relatives of substance abusers
tel: 071-731 8060
5-7 Parsons Green,
London, SW6 4UL

Mainliners
Drug users with HIV
P.O. Box 125,

London, SW9 8EF

RELEASE
Drug problems and legal
  consequences
tel: 071-377 5905/603 8654
  (24 hours)
169 Commercial Street,
London, E1 6BW

RESOLVE
Advice on local counselling for
  stopping sniffing glue, solvents or
  gas
tel: 0785 817885

SCODA
Information, help and advice on
  drugs
tel: 071-430 2341

TRANX
Broad range of help for tranquilliser
  users
tel: 081-427 2065/2847 (24 hours)
25A Masons Avenue,
Wealdstone,
Harrow,
Middlesex, HA3 5AH

Turning Point
Help with drugs and alcohol abuse,
  including residential homes and
  training courses
tel: 071-606 3947
4th Floor, CAP House,
9-12 Long Lane,
London, EC1A 9HA

Elderly
Age Concern
tel: 081-640 5431
Age Concern England,
Bernard Sunley House,
60 Pitcairn Road,
Mitcham,
Surrey, CR4 3LL

Anchor Housing
Provides sheltered housing for the
   elderly and general advice on
   accommodation problems
tel: 0865 722261
Oxenford House,
13–15 Magdalen Street,
Oxford, OX1 3BP

Contact
Group for isolated elderly people
tel: 071-240 0630
15 Henrietta Street,
London, WC2E 8QH

Counsel and Care for the Elderly
tel: 071-485 1550
16 Bonny Street,
London, NW1 9TG

Over-Sixties Employment Bureau
tel: 071-703 5066
186 Crampton Street,
London, SE17 3AE

Family Planning
Brook Advisory Centres
tel: 071-323 1522
233 Tottenham Court Road,
London, W1P 9AE

Family Planning Association
tel: 071-636 7866
27–35 Mortimer Street,
London, W1N 7RJ

See telephone directory for local
   family planning clinics.

Gambling
Gam-anon
tel: 071-352 3060

**General Dental and Medical
   Practitioners**
For lists of practitioners in your area
   contact:

- Family Practitioner Committee
   (FPC) (found in local
   telephone directory)
- Your local main general post
   office

Health Education
Health Education Authority —
   advice on local Health Education
   Departments
tel: 071-631 0930
Hamilton House,
Mabledon Place,
London, WC1H 9TX

Also see local telephone directory.

Hearing Problems
British Association for the Hard of
   Hearing
tel: 081-743 1110/1353
7–11 Armstrong Road,
London, W3 7JL

British Deaf Association
tel: 0228 48844
Prestel: 022848844; Telecom Gold:
   79BKU44
38 Victoria Place,
Carlisle, CA1 1HLL

National Deaf-blind and Rubella
   Association
tel: 071-278 1005
311 Gray's Inn Road,
London, WC1X 8PT

National Deaf Children's Society
tel: 071-229 9272
45 Hereford Road,
London, W2 5AH

Homosexuality
Lesbian Line
tel: 071-251 6911
Box BM 1514
London, WC1N 3XX

London Lesbian and Gay
  Switchboard
tel: 071-837 7324
BM Switchboard,
London, WC1N 3XX

Marital Problems
Divorce Conciliation Advisory
  Service
tel: 071-730 2422
38 Ebury Street,
London, SW1 0LU

National Council for the Divorced
  and Separated
tel: 0533 708880 (24 hours)
13 High Street,
Little Shelford,
Cambridge, CB2 5ES

National Family Conciliation Council
tel: 0793 618486
34 Milton Street,
Swindon,
Wiltshire, SN1 5JA

Relate (formerly Marriage Guidance
  Council) Look in 'phone book
  under either 'M' or 'R'

Medical Conditions
Alzheimer's Disease Society
tel: 081-675 6557/8/9
158-60 Balham High Road,
London, SW12 9BN

Arthritis Care,
tel: 071-235 0902
6 Grosvenor Crescent,
London, SW1X 7ER

Association for Spina Bifida (ASBAH)
tel: 071-388 1382
22 Upper Woburn Place,
London, WC1H 0EP

Asthma Society
tel: 071-226 2260

300 Upper Street,
London, N1 2XX

Bechet's Syndrome Society
tel: 0904 37310
3 Belgrave Street,
Haxby Road,
York, YO3 7YY

Breastcare and Mastectomy
  Association
tel: 071-837 0908
26 Harrison Street,
London, WC1H 8JG

Brent Sickle Cell Centre
tel: 081-459 1292 Ext. 4235
Willesden General Hospital
Harlesden Road,
London, NW10 3RY

British Association of Cancer
  Patients
tel: 071-608 1785
121-123 Charterhouse Street,
London, EC1M 6AA

British Diabetic Association
tel: 071-323 1531
10 Queen Ann Street,
London, W1M 0BD

British Dyslexia Association
tel: 0734 668271
98 London Road,
Reading, RG1 5AU

British Epilepsy Association
tel: 0532 439393
Anstey House,
40 Hanover Square,
Leeds, LS3 1BE

British Kidney Patient Association
tel: 04203 2022
Bordon,
Hampshire, GU35 9JP

British Migraine Association

tel: 09323 52468
178A High Road,
Byfleet,
Weybridge,
Surrey, KT14 7ED

Cancer Contact
tel: 07918 4754
6 Meadows,
Hassocks,
West Sussex

Cancerlink — information on all
   aspects of cancer
tel: 071-833 2451
46 Pentonville Road,
London, N1 9HF

Chest, Heart and Stroke Association
tel: 071-387 3012
Tavistock House North,
Tavistock Square,
London, WC1H 9JE

Coeliac Society of the UK
tel: 0494 37278
P.O. Box 220,
High Wycombe,
Bucks, HP11 2HY

Colostomy Welfare Group,
tel: 071-828 5175
38–39 Eccleston Square,
London, SW1V 1PB

Cystic Fibrosis Research Trust
tel: 081-464 7211/2
Alexandra House,
5 Blythe Road,
Bromley,
Kent, BR1 3RS

Diabetic Foundation
tel: 081-656 5467
177A Tennison Road,
London, SE25 5N

Down's Syndrome Association
tel: 071-720 0008

12–13 Clapham Common Southside,
London, SW4 7AA

Friedrich's Ataxia Group
tel: 0483 272741
The Common,
Cranleigh,
Surrey, GU6 8SB

Haemophilia Society
tel: 071-928 2020
123 Westminster Bridge Road,
London, SE1 7HR

Ileostomy Association
tel: 0623 28099
Ambleshurt House,
Black Scotch Lane,
Mansfield,
Notts, NG1 4PF

Leukaemia Research Fund
tel: 071-405 0101
43 Great Ormond Street,
London, WC1N 3JJ

Leukaemia Care Society
tel: 0392 218514
P.O. Box 82,
Exeter,
Devon, EX2 5DP

Mastectomy Association
tel: 071-837 0908
26 Harrison Street,
London, WC1H 8JG

Motor Neurone Disease Association
tel: 0604 250505/22269
61 Derngate,
Northampton, NN1 1VE

Multiple Sclerosis Society
tel: 071-736 6267
25 Effie Road,
London, SW6 1EE

Myalgic Encephalomyelitis (ME)
   Association

tel: 03756 42466
P.O. Box 8,
Stanford-le-Hope,
Sussex, SS17 8EX

National Association for Colitis and
Crohn's Disease
tel: 0727 44296
98A London Road,
St Albans,
Herts, AL1 1NX

National Autistic Society
tel: 081-451 3844
276 Willesden Lane,
London, NW2 5RB

National Back Pain Association
tel: 081-977 5474
31–33 Park Road,
Teddington,
Middlesex, TW11 0AB

Parkinson's Disease Society
tel: 071-255 2432
36 Portland Place,
London, W1N 3DG

Psoriasis Association
tel: 0604 711129
7 Milton Street,
Northampton, NN2 7JG

Renal Society
tel: 071-485 9775
41 Mutton Place,
London, NW1 8DF

Sickle Cell Society
tel: 081-961 7795
Green Lodge,
Barretts Green Road,
London, W10 7AP

Sole Mates — to help people with
different sized feet to make the
necessary contacts
tel: 081-524 2423
46 Gordon Road,

Chingford,
London, E4 6BU

Spastic Society
tel: 071-636 5020
12 Park Crescent,
London, W1N 4EQ

Spinal Injuries Association
tel: 081-444 2121
Yeoman House,
76 St James' Lane,
London, N10 3DF

UK Thalassaemia Society
tel: 081-348 0437
107 Nightingale Lane,
London, N8 7QY

Mental Handicap
British Institute of Mental Handicap
tel: 0562 850251
Wolverhampton Road,
Kidderminster,
Worcs., DY10 3PP

Mencap — help for mentally
handicapped adults and children
tel: 071-253 9433
123 Golden Lane,
London, EC1Y 0RH

MIND — National Association for
Mental Health
Day care, sheltered employment,
housing
tel: 071-637 0741
22 Harley Street,
London, W1N 2ED

Scottish Down's Syndrome
Association
tel: 031-226 2420
54 Shandwick Place,
Edinburgh, EH2 4RT

Scottish Society for the Mentally
Handicapped

tel: 041-226 4541
13 Elmbank Street,
Glasgow G2 4AQ

Psychiatric Illness
Anorexic Aid — self-help groups
Local Branches
tel: 0494 21431

Anorexic Aid
The Priory Centre,
11 Priory Road,
High Wycombe,
Bucks, HP13 6SL

Bulimia and Anorexia Nervosa
  Group
tel: 0253 726829
27 Lawrence Avenue,
Lytham St Anne's,
Lancs, FY8 3LG

MIND
tel: 071-637 0741
22 Harley Street,
London, W1N 2ED

National Schizophrenia Fellowship
tel: 081-390 3651
78 Victoria Road,
Surbiton,
Surrey, KT6 4NS

Psychotherapy
British Association of
  Psychotherapists
Non-NHS. Low-cost.
tel: 081-346 1747
121 Hendon Lane,
London, N3 3PR

London Clinic of Psychoanalysis
Non-NHS. Low-cost.
63 New Cavendish Street,
London, W1M 7RD
tel: 071-580 4952

Tavistock Clinic — NHS

tel: 071-435 7111
Belsize Lane,
London, NW3 5BA

Women's Therapy Centre
Help with stress and eating
  disorders, etc.
tel: 071-263 6200
6 Manor Gardens,
London, N7 6LA

Rape
Rape Crisis Centre
tel: 071-278 3956/837 1600
P.O. Box 69,
London, WC1X 9NJ

Retirement
Pre-Retirement Association
tel: 081-767 3225/6
19 Undine Street,
London, SW17 8PP

REACH — Retired Executives Action
  Clearing House
Information on available voluntary
  work
89 Southwark Street,
London, SE1 0HD

Single Parents
National Council for One-Parent
  Families
tel: 071-267 1361
255 Kentish Town Road,
London, NW5 2LX

Scottish Council for Single Parents
tel: 031-556 3899
13 Gayfield Square,
Edinburgh, EH1 3NX

Smoking
ASH — Action on Smoking and
  Health
tel: 071-637 9843/6

5–11 Mortimer Street,
London, W1N 7RH

Health Education Authority
Will supply leaflets on giving up
    smoking, and information on
    support agencies.
Hamilton House,
Mabledon Place,
London, WC1H 9TX

Quitline
tel: 071-323 0505
Will give information about local
    sources of help for giving up
    smoking.

Women's Problems — Social and
    Medical
London Women's Aid
Help with temporary
    accommodation for women and
    children in crisis due to physical
    and mental violence
tel: 071-251 6537

52–54 Featherstone Street,
London, EC1Y 8RT

National Council for Women
tel: 071-354 2395
36 Danbury Street,
London, N1 8JU

The British Menopause Society
tel: 0628 890199
83 High Street,
Marlow,
Bucks, SL7 1AB

Women's Nutritional Advisory
    Service and PMT Advisory Service
tel: 0273 771366
P.O. Box 268,
Hove,
East Sussex, BN3 1RW

Working Mothers Association
tel: 071-700 5771
77 Holloway Road,
London, N7 8JZ

Health and Safety Executive (HSE) publications relevant to health care work

The HSE is responsible to the Health and Safety Commission — a government sponsored body made up of representatives from the Trades Union Congress, Confederation of British Industry, universities and local authorities. Its publications are obtainable from:

Her Majesty's Stationery Office Books, PO Box 276, London, SW8 5DT.

and the following government bookshops:

London	● 49 High Holborn, WC1V 6HB (callers only) Tel: 071-873 0011
	● PO Box 276, SW8 5DT. Tel: 071-873 9090 (telephone orders only)
Edinburgh	● EH3 9AZ: HMSO Books, 71 Lothian Road. Tel: 031-453 4181
Manchester	● M60 8AS: 9–21 Princess Street. Tel: 061-834 7201
Bristol	● BS1 2BQ: Southey House, Wine Street. Tel: 0272 24306/24307
Birmingham	● B1 2HE: 258 Broad Street. Tel: 021-643 3740
Belfast	● BT1 4JY: 80 Chicester Street. Tel: 0232 238451

Publications are also obtainable from booksellers acting as agents for Her Majesty's Stationery Office.

ACGM/HSE/Notes

ACGM/HSE/NOTE 7
Guidelines for the categorization of genetic manipulation experiments, (1988).

ACGM/HSE/NOTE 8
Laboratory containment facilities for genetic manipulation, (1988).

Health and Safety Commission Leaflets

HSC 11
Health and safety at Work etc. Act 1974: your obligations to non-employees, (1985).

Health and Safety Executive Leaflets

HSE 11 (rev)
Reporting an injury or a dangerous occurrence, (1986).

HSE 17
Reporting a case of disease: a brief guide to the Reporting of Injuries, Diseases and Dangerous Occurrences Regulations 1985, (1986).

HSE 21
Report that accident: RIDDOR The Reporting of Injuries, Diseases and Dangerous Occurrences Regulations 1985 (1988).

Health Hazard Information Sheets

Health hazard information sheet 5: solvents. rev., (1988)
Health hazard information sheet 6: AIDS, (1987).
Health hazard information sheet 7: skin hazards, (1987).

IAC (Industry Advisory Committee) Leaflets

IAC/L5
Asbestos hazard in health service buildings (pocket card issued by Health Services Advisory Committee), (1983).

IAC/L22
AIDS: prevention of infection in the health services, (1986).

IND(G) Leaflets

IND(G)4rev(P)
First aid at work: general guidance for inclusion in first aid boxes, (1987).

IND(G)36(L)
Working with VDUs, (1986).

IND(G)54(L)
Asbestos: does your company work with asbestos? (1988).

IND(G)58(L)
Review your occupational health needs: employer's checklist, (1988).

IND(G)59(L)
Mental health at work, (1988).

IND(G)63(L)
Passive smoking at work, (1988).

IND(G)65(L)
Introducing COSHH: a brief guide for all employers to the new requirements, (1988).

IND(G)66(L)
VCM and you. Control of Substances Hazardous to Health Regulations 1988 (COSHH), (1988).

IND(G)67(L)
Hazard and risk explained. Control of Substances Hazardous to Health Regulations 1988 (COSHH), (1988).

IND(S) Leaflets

IND(S)9(L)
Wear your film badge, (1984).

IND(S)23(C)
Asbestos: new asbestos regulations, (1988).

Medical Advice

M50
Ionizing Radiations Regulations 1985: applying for a review of a medical decision, (1986).

Medical Series Leaflets

MS(B)6(rev)
Save your skin: occupational contact dermatitis, (1987).

MS(B)10
Save your skin: wear gloves, (1987). (Available from Employment Medical Advisory Services in HSE Area Offices and HSE Public Enquiry Points)

PL

PL 811 (free)
AIDS. Acquired immune deficiency syndrome and employment. Department of Employment/HSE, (1986). (Available from The Mailing House, Leeland Road, London W13 9HL)

Specialist Inspector Reports

SIR10
Sick building syndrome: a review, by J. M. Sykes, (1988).

SIR11
Precautions against illness associated with humidifiers, by J. M. Sykes, (1988).

Advisory and Joint Standing Committee Reports

Dangerous Pathogens, Advisory Committee on categorization of pathogens according to hazard and categories of containment, (1984).

Guidance on the use testing and maintenance of laboratory and animal flexible film isolators, (1985).

Inactivation of viral haemorrhagic fever specimens with B-propiolactone, (1988).

LAV/HTLV III — the causative agent of AIDS and related conditions: revised guidelines, (1986).

Genetic Manipulation, Advisory Committee on

ACGM/HSE/NOTE 1 (revision)
Guidance on construction of recombinants containing potentially oncogenic nucleic acid sequences, (1987).

ACGM/HSE/NOTE 4

Guidelines for the health surveillance of those involved in genetic manipulation at laboratory and large scale, (1986).

ACGM/HSE/NOTE 6
Guidelines for the large-scale use of genetically manipulated organisms, (1987).

ACGM/HSE/NOTE 7
Guidelines for the categorization of genetic manipulation experiments, (1988).

ACGM/HSE/NOTE 8
Laboratory containment facilities for genetic manipulation, (1988).

Guidance on the recording of accidents and incidents in the health services, (1986).

Guidelines on occupational health services in the health services, (1984).

Lifting of patients in the health services, (1984).

List of guidance on health, safety and welfare in the health service, (1984).

Safe disposal of clinical waste, (1982).

Safety in health service laboratories: Hepatitis B precautions to minimize the risk of infection from specimens known or suspected to be positive and in the testing of specimens for the presence of hepatitis B antigens or antibodies, (1985).

Safety in health service laboratories: the labelling, transport and reception of specimens, (1986).

Safety policies in the health service, (1983).

Violence to staff in the health services, (1987).

Approved and Other Codes of Practice

Approved Codes of Practice Issued Under Section 16 of the Health and Safety at Work Etc Act 1974

COP 16
Protection of persons against ionizing radiation arising from

any work activity: The Ionizing Radiations Regulations 1985: approved code of practice, (1985).

Health effects of VDUs : A Bibliography (1984).

Guidance Notes

Environmental Hygiene

EH 17
Mercury — health and safety precautions, (1977).

EH 26
Occupational skin diseases: health and safety precautions, (1981).

Medical Series

MS 21
Precautions for the safe handling of cytotoxic drugs, (1983).

Plant and Machinery

PM 8
Passenger–carrying paternosters, (1977).

Health and Safety: Guidance Booklets

HS(G)20
Guidelines for occupational health services, (1980).

Health and Safety: Regulations Booklets

HS(R)11
First aid at work, (1981).

HS(R)12
Guide to the Health and Safety (Dangerous Pathogens) Regulations 1981, (1981).

HS(R)16
Guide to the Notification of Installations Handling Hazardous Substances Regulations 1982, (1983).

HS(R)23
Guide to the Reporting of Injuries, Diseases and Dangerous Occurrences Regulations 1985, (1986).

IND(G) Leaflets

IND(G)4Rev(P)
First aid at work: general guidance for inclusion in first aid boxes, (1987).

IND(G)57(L)
Review your occupational health needs: employers guide, (1988).

IND(G)59(L)
Mental health at work, (1988).

Toxicity Reviews

TR 2
Formaldehyde, (1981).

Unnumbered Reports

COSHH assessments: a step by step guide to assessment and the skills needed for it. Control of Substances Hazardous to Health Regulations 1988, (1988).

Genetic manipulation (regulations and guidance notes) 1978.

Handbook of radiological protection (Part 1, data), (1971 O/P).

Preventing violence to staff (B. Poyner and C. Warne. HSE/Tavistock Institute of Human Relations) 1988.

Protection against ionizing radiations in medical and dental practice, (1988).

Research and Laboratory Services Division of the Health and Safety Executive: an account of the Health and Safety Executive's research testing and scientific support services, (1983).

Safe disposal of clinical waste, (1982).

Some aspects of noise and hearing loss: notes on the problem of noise at work and report of the HSE Working Group on machinery noise, (1981 O/P).

Statement of policy for the development of occupational health services, by the Chairman of the Health and Safety Commission, Dr. J. Cullen, (1986).

Violence to staff: a basis for assessment and prevention (B. Poyner and C. Warne, Tavistock Institute of Human Relation), (1986).

Visual display units, (1983).

Watch your step: prevention of slipping, tripping and falling accidents at work, (1985).

Writing your health and safety policy statement, (1986).

Bibliography

The following is a list of books which might form the basis of a library in an occupational health department. It is not intended to be exhaustive.

Adams, R. M. (ed.), (1990). *Occupational Skin Disease*, 2nd ed., Philadelphia: W. B. Saunders.

Advisory Committee on Dangerous Pathogens, (1984). *Categorization of Pathogens According to Hazard and Categories of Containment*, London: Department of Health.

Advisory Committee on Dangerous Pathogens, (1990). *HIV — The Causative Agent of AIDS and Related Condition. Second Revision of Guidelines*, London: Department of Health.

British Medical Association, (1987). *Immunization Against Hepatitis B*, London: BMA.

British Medical Association, (1989). *A Code of Practice for Sterilization of Instruments and Control of Cross Infection*. London: BMA.

British Medical Association (1990). *A Code of Practice for the Safe Use and Disposal of Sharps*. London: BMA.

Brune, D. K., Edling, C. (eds.), (1989). *Occupational Hazards in the Health Professions*, Boca Baton: CRC Press.

Cotes, J. E., Steel, J. (1987). *Work-related Lung Disorders*, Oxford: Blackwell Scientific.

Edwards, F. C., McCallum, R. I., Taylor, P. J. (eds.), (1988). *Fitness for work. The Medical Aspect*, Oxford: OUP.

Expert Advisory Group on AIDS, (1990). *Guidance for Clinical*

Health Care Workers: Protection Against Infection with HIV and Hepatitis Viruses, London: HMSO.

Harris, C. J. (ed.), (1984). *Occupational Health Nursing Practice*, Bristol: Wright.

Howard, J. K., Tyrer, F. H. (eds.), (1987). *Textbook of Occupational Medicine*, London: Churchill Livingstone.

Joint Committee on Vaccination and Immunisation, (1990). *Immunisation Against Infectious Diseases*, London: HMSO.

Klaassen, C. D., Amdur, M. O., Doull, J. (eds.), (1986). *Casarett and Doull's toxicology*, 3rd edn., New York: McMillan.

Liberman, D. F., Gordon, J. G. (eds.), (1989). *Biohazards Management Handbook*, New York: Marcel Dekker.

London Waste Authority, (1989). *Guidelines for the Segregation, Handling and Transport of Clinical Waste*, London: LWA.

Lowbury, E. J. L., Ayliffe, G. A. J., Geddes, A. M., *et al.* (eds.), (1981). *Control of Hospital Infection. A Practical Handbook*, 2nd edn., London: Chapman and Hall.

Parkes, R. (1985). *Occupational Lung Disorders*, 2nd edn., London: Butterworths.

Payne, R., Firth-Cozens, J. (eds.) (1987). *Stress in Health Professionals*, Chichester: John Wiley.

Raffle, P. A. B., Lee, W. R., McCallum, R. I., *et al.* (eds.), (1987). *Hunter's Diseases of Occupations*, London: Hodder and Stoughton.

Rom, W. N. (ed.), (1983). *Environmental and Occupational Medicine*, Boston: Little Brown.

Slaney, B. (ed.), (1980). *Occupational Health Nursing*, London: Croom Helm.

Subcommittee of the Joint Tuberculosis Committee of the British Thoracic Society, (1990). Control and prevention of tuberculosis in Britain: an update of the code of practice, Br. Med. J., **300**, 995–999.

United States Department of Health and Human Services (1988). *Guidelines for Protecting the Safety and Health of Health Care*

Workers. DHHS (NIOSH) Publication No 88–119. Washington: US Government Printing Office.

Waldron, H. A. (ed.), (1989) *Occupational Health Practice,* 3rd edn., London: Butterworths.

Waldron, H. A. (1990). *Lecture Notes on Occupational Medicine,* 4th edn., Oxford: Blackwell Scientific.

Zenz, C. (ed.), (1988). *Occupational Medicine. Principles and Practical Applications,* 2nd edn., Chicago: Year Book, Medical Publishers.

Index

staff shortages 5
stress 3
pregnancy, *see* pregnancy
standardized mortality ratios
32
health surveillance:
lasers 59–60
radio-isotopes 56–7
routine 30–31
hepatitis B, 33–4, 75–9
hepatitis C 34
herpes simplex virus 38, 88
herpetic whitlow 108
human immunodeficiency virus
(HIV) 80–82, 118
hygienist 20, 50

infection control policies 65
infections:
enteric 86–7
haemolytic streptococcal 38,
87, 107–8
staphylococcal 87–8, 107–9
viral 38
wound 87
infectious diseases 32–6, 38
exposure during pregnancy
117–18
job risk to hospital staff 28
influenza 88–9
ionizing radiation *see* radiation

laboratory staff:
causes of accidents 100
chest X-rays 30–31
hepatitis B risk 75
lasers 57–60
lifting:
and back pain 61, 110–13
as cause of back injuries 100
pregnancy 115
techniques, training 18
litigation, release of occupational
health records 10

managers, hospital:
communication with 5, 9
notification of an applicant's
fitness for work 11–12,
30
Mantoux test 35, 71–2
medical students 75–6, 127
meningococcal meningitis 38,
79–80
mental illness 10, 18, 124–6
mercury 46–7, 51
methylene chloride 49

needlestick injuries, *see* sharps
injuries
nitrous oxide 44
noise 64
nurses *see* health service staff,
nurses; practitioners, nurses

occupational health department:
accommodation 6–7
central monitoring of sickness
absence rates 94–5
composition of staff 17
contacts with outside agencies
18–20
management 7–8
records 9–11, 102
as source of information 13
training budget 21
occupational health practitioners,
see practitioners
occupational health service:
doctors' attitudes 120–21
economics 4–5
ethics 10
provided for non-health
service staff 13–15
staffing 16–21
workload increased by COSHH
regulations 31
occupational health training
20–21, 127
occupational hygienist 20, 50